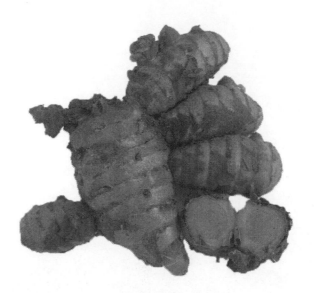

Turmeric

The Ayurvedic
Spice of Life

Prashanti de Jager
MSc, EMT

PIØNEER
IMPRINTS

second edition, 2010

vidyasagar publications
in conjunction with pioneer imprints

www.pioneerimprints.com

book design: alden bevington
cover design: d. l. frazer

isbn: 978-0-9818318-9-3

cataloging-in-publication data available upon request.

note: this book is a work in progress and is being updated steadily.
If you have any comments or suggestions please feel free to contact the
author at:

www.prashantidejager.com

Disclaimer

Few of the scientific tests to prove the benefits of turmeric are directly referenced here. One reason for this is that I believe that all the claims have been proven beyond the shadow of a doubt in a test which has lasted at least 6000 years and which included literally billions of people of all ages. The test that I am speaking about is the Ayurvedic tradition of India.

This book contains as much about my peregrinations of India, Nepal, and the stacks of Herb libraries such as the one at UC Davis, as it does theactual information I found in these sources. Feel free to have fun, taking the actual folklore with a grain of salt and the science with a pinch of Turmeric.

Footnotes are not used to indicate the source of laboratory and clinical finding. Rather the bibliography is organized by topic so that you can peruse the literature of your particular interest. There are about 500 scientific references listed here as of 1997. Now that list would be closer to 5000. Contact me if you are interested in that list.

Acknowledgements

This Book is Dedicated to Allies

This book is about acknowledging a great ally, Turmeric, and before the story begins I would like to acknowledge some other wonderful allies which have made the publication possible. For over 4 decades Gregory Masck continues to be an epic ally and constant rooted source of Love and Support to me, unbelievably so. Alden Bevington of Pioneer Imprints is a key ally in many respects who designed both the book and much of its trajectory. D.L. Frazer (sweetanomaly@gmail.com) designed the cover layers and brings an important aspect of family to the project. Shekhar Malhotra of Full Circle is a veritable gateway who immensely amplifies what goodness gets cultured across the planet. Gratitude so naturally renders me when I even think of these allies and all the others. Thank you so. Om

Table of Contents

Foreword, by Dr. David Frawley

If I had only a single herb to depend upon for all possible health and dietary needs, I would without much hesitation choose the Indian spice turmeric. There is little that it cannot do in the realm of healing and much that no other herb is able to accomplish. Turmeric has a broad spectrum of actions, mild but certain effects, and is beneficial for long term and daily usage. Though it is a common spice, few people, including herbalists know of its great value and are using it to the extent possible. It is an herb that one should get to know and live with.

Turmeric is best known as an excellent spice for East Indian cooking. It is the basis of most Indian curries, which traditionally are composed of at least half of it, giving them their characteristic yellow color. The herb itself has a mild spicy yet slightly bitter taste that deepens the natural taste of food and is not too hot for those sensitive to chilies or other strongly aromatic spices. Turmeric helps balance the effects of other spices, blending their tastes and properties in a synergistic manner, giving them a better flavor.

Turmeric gently stimulates the digestive fire and makes the food easier to digest and absorb. It also helps detoxify the food, killing bacteria and even parasites that may be found within it. In addition it improves the quality of food, adding nutritive and blood building properties to the oils with which it combines, particularly ghee (clarified butter), with which it has an important affinity. It is essential to Ayurvedic diets and a helpful aid to any gourmet cooking.

Yet turmeric is also an excellent herb for first aid and for injuries of all types, both acute and chronic. It is a mild astringent that is marvelous applied externally for all kinds of cuts, wounds, bruises and soft tissue damage. It helps stop bleeding and improve healing, clearing out dead and damaged tissue and promoting the growth of new healthy cells. There are many miraculous stories about how fresh turmeric used on severe cuts or wounds has allowed them to heal without scars. The powder is good for first aid and should be part of any herbal first aid kit. The herb is excellent post-surgery for promoting healing and preventing the formation of scar tissue. Its astringent properties make it an excellent gargle for sore throats and cough, for which it is taken with a little salt.

In addition turmeric is a great woman's herb and is helpful for many gynecological problems. It mildly promotes menstruation, relieves menstrual pain and cramping, is great for countering PMS, and helps build the blood. It helps guard against or even remove cysts in the breast or uterus, and is a good guard against breast cancer. It helps strengthen the female reproductive organs and aid in their proper formation in young women, while helping soothing and harmonizing the body during menopause. In addition it helps beautify the skin and improve the complexion, promoting circulation and nutrition to the surface of the body.

Turmeric is an important herb for the heart and the liver. It strengthens the heart, helping lower cholesterol and preventing heart disease, strokes and heart attacks. It is a mild blood thinner that has no side effects and does not cause anemia. It cleanses the liver and gently promotes the flow of bile, relieving emotional tension and depression, and clearing out toxins, including pollutants and chemicals of various types from deep within the body. It helps counters addictions to alcohol and to sugar. It is especially good for diabetes and can prevent or control adult onset diabetes if taken on a regular basis with meals.

Perhaps most importantly today in the age of immune system disorders turmeric is an excellent adaptogen and tonic. It promotes healing on all levels of the body-mind, stimulates proper tissue formation, aids in rejuvenation and increases longevity. It helps with weak immune conditions, chronic fevers, and even seemingly intractable and incurable diseases like Cancer and Aids. It helps dissolve blood stagnation, break up tumors, and eliminates cysts of all kinds. It is a natural regulator for optimal health and energy.

Ayurvedically speaking turmeric works well on all the doshas. Its taste and action is particularly anti-Kapha, reducing mucus and fat from the system. As a mild and not too hot spice even Pitta types can take it, particularly along with bitters or cool spices like coriander, which makes it a good liver tonic for them. Vata types can also benefit from it, particularly as taken with food or with other herbal tonics.

Turmeric works well in combination with many other herbs, which serve to bring out its different properties. For the liver it works well with bitters like aloe, gentian and barberry. For the heart it synergizes with heart tonics like guggul or arjuna. For female problems it works well with emmenagogues like dan gui or myrrh. For digestion it combines well with ginger and cardamom.

For all these reasons turmeric is likened to the Divine Mother, bestowing numerous blessings and helping us in all dangers, difficulties and conditions of weakness and debility. It vitalizes the body's own natural healing energy through its action of strengthening digestion and circulation, and aiding in the regulation of all bodily systems. That it can be taken as a spice or along with food makes it much easier to use as well.

It is apt therefore that turmeric at last has its own book, which is long overdue. Just as turmeric is like a pharmacopoeia in itself, it deserves its own extended study and treatise. Prashanti de Jager has done an excellent job revealing the secrets of this great herb and its many properties and various levels of action. There is nothing like it in the literature about the herb. Nor do we find similar Ayurvedic studies of other herbs. Prashanti has examined turmeric both from traditional Ayurvedic and modern scientific accounts, going into great detail about its properties. He has added many interesting case studies that highlight the herb's power and show its relevance. Notably he has covered the entire field of the herb's many properties and applications.

"Turmeric, the Ayurvedic Spice of Life", should be part of the library of every herbalist or anyone interested in plants and spices. Turmeric is indeed the spice of life. It carries the energy of life to our entire being and connects us to the beneficent forces of this conscious universe in which we live. It is also perhaps the most useful, and certainly the most commonly used Ayurvedic herb. Turmeric is a good place to start studying and using Ayurveda and a good herb with which to take a new lease on life.

Dr. David Frawley (Vamadeva Shastri)
Author, *Yoga and Ayurveda: Self-Healing and Self-Realization*,
***Ayurvedic Healing*, etc.**

I

Turmeric: An Introduction

The human body is a very rare gift of nature.
Take very good care of your body and mind,
don't put the Diamond in a plastic bag.

The worst pollution to the body is bad thoughts
and the worst thought is "I am the body."
Your diet is also important so eat sattvic food.
Simple food cooked with Love and eaten with friends
is tastiest of all.

To be healed first you must decide
that you want to be free of pain and suffering.
Without wanting this nothing else will work.

Sri H. W. L. Poonja

Great Healers! In one form or another they are sought out by all of us. Somewhere inside we all seek balanced happy lives and so we seek that which will grant us health and joy. This book is about Turmeric, one of the planets great healers. This healer is not obscured in some esoterica and not distanced by a cosmic price tag. As usual with great healers it is very close to you and readily accessible, in fact, it is probably in your house right now.

13

Good fortune has allowed me to study Turmeric and many other great Ayurvedic herbs for the last 10 years. I lived in India from 1990 to 1997 learning the essence of the Vedic Tradition, of which Ayurveda is a part. I studied with dozens of teachers and Gurus from all over the awesome continent from the high Himalayas to the northern plains, through the jungles of central India to the ancient Dravidian Mountains of Tamil Nadu and the friendly coasts of Kerala. My SatGuru is Sri H.W.L. Poonja of Lucknow, a disciple of Sri Ramana Maharishi of Tiruvannamalai.

Before leaving for India I spent 6 years studying several different Healing traditions in Ann Arbor, Michigan, where I also received a M.S. from the University of Michigan. One day I just could not fight the pull to India anymore and so I left everything and flew to England, where I started an overland journey of amazement to Mother India and then throughout her endless 'States' and experiences. Cold intellectual facts do not interest me anymore. To me experience is more attractive and so it is from and with my experience of India's treasures that this book is offered to you.

As I wander through India one of the most common sights, or should I say sensations, is that of Turmeric. Perhaps the most common sight of turmeric is red turmeric, kumkum, which is typically Turmeric and/or Saffron and/or the fruit of the Sindhur Tree mixed with lime (calcium hydroxide) to turn it red. Kumkum is worn as a tilak, the red dot between the eyes of most Hindu women and many of the men. The Tilak symbolizes several things from marriage to dedication to God. I am sure it also serves as medicine as the third eye is such a sensitive place and hence a great location to apply an herb. Perhaps kumkum filters third eye perceptions. Perhaps it helps keep the sinuses clear. Perhaps it protects one from negative influences. Perhaps it is just the ritual of applying it, and the keeping of the object of devotion in your mind is the real medicine.

Yellow faced women are a common sight in the Indian bazaar. Apply to your face a layer of a paste made of turmeric with milk or water and you have one of the planet's great facials. The downside of this to most westerners is then you also have a yellow face for a couple of days, but this doesn't stop the average Indian woman who has no problem shopping the bazaars while looking like she has just powdered gold dust onto her face. I really appreciate this attitude more and more as I awaken to the friendly protection offered by this earthy herb of the Sun.

Assuming you spend more time outside than in restaurants, the next most common sight of Turmeric is in the food. It is practically everywhere and given that there are almost a billion people in India, it is not an exaggeration to say that at least 700 million people there eat 2 or 3 grams of Turmeric everyday.

Walking through the bazaars you are bound to find a masala wallah, a spice seller, with mounds of turmeric which he is selling by the kilo. It is a great sight in the midst of mountains of clove buds and black pepper fruits, amla berries and coriander seeds, cinnamon bark and cardamom pods and all these marvelous colorful spices that we take for granted everyday. I love to sit with the sellers and talk about where the spices come from, what seasons are best for what, and what the herbs and spices are used for medicinally. They know all the folk cures and are a great source of information. Ayurveda is as full of commonsense as it is humming of the mystical and so it is with the common people of India, like the spice sellers and the village mothers, that so much of Ayurveda is learned and passed on from elder to child for countless generations. In this way the ability of Turmeric is proven and its legacy grows. I have learned so much from them that I could never have learned elsewhere. This is confirmed by Paracelcus who in 1493 wrote:

"The physician does not learn everything he must know and Master from a high college alone. From time to time he must consult old women, gypsies, magicians, wayfarers and all manner of peasant folk and random people and learn from them, for these people have more knowledge about such things than all the high colleges."

Outer Beauty, Inner Purity. This is what Turmeric gives to us. Used on a daily basis for thousands of years in India by most of its population it is traditionally considered to have dozens of beneficial properties. What Ayurveda has known for millennium modern science is now starting to prove for itself in laboratories and clinics around the world. Turmeric improves liver and heart function, helps with arthritis and diabetes, and attacks cancer and carcinogens. You will also notice the difference it makes with your skin. Beautiful clarity.

Most of the Ayurvedic doctors that I meet in India consider turmeric, or Haldi, as it is known in Hindi, to be one of the best herbs of India, and some go as far saying that it is the best. Sourcing from my own experiences, from traditional wisdom in the form of Ayurvedic doctors, spice sellers, and Mothers, and from contemporary scientific reports I would like to present to you some of my notes regarding this great herb.

2

Turmeric: A Medical Summary

The authority of hundreds of scientific articles from reliable sources, thousands of years of daily use, and millions of people around the planet establishes the following properties and uses of Turmeric, her essential oils, her water soluble extracts and her curcumins.

Healing Properties of Turmeric

The following list describes the traditional uses of Turmeric. On the next page a more exhaustive list is given that describes the healing properties intrinsic to Turmeric from a western pharmacology point of view.

Alterative *Restores normal functioning of organ systems*
Analgesic *Relieves pain*
Antibacterial *Antibiotic, reduces and destroys pathogenic bacteria*
Anti inflammatory *Counteracts inflammation and its effects*
Anti-tumor *Prevents and treats tumor and cancer*
Anti-allergic *Helps normalize the immune system*
Antioxidant *Inhibits oxidation and cellular aging*
Antiseptic *Inhibits both local and systemic infections*
Antispasmodic *Relieves spasms*

Astringent   *Brings firmness back to tissue, reduces discharges*
Cardiovascular   *Is a tonic to the heart*
Carminative   *Soothes the digestive tract, removes gas*
Cholagogue   *Stimulates liver/gall bladder*
Digestive   *Normalizes digestive capacity*
Stimulant   *Moves the energy*
Vulnerary   *Wound healing*

Selected Therapeutic Uses of Turmeric

Aids/HIV	*Indigestion*
Anemia	*Irritable Bowel Syndrome*
Cancer	*Parasites*
Diabetes	*Poor Circulation*
Digestion	*Staph Infections*
Female Regulator	*Skin Disorders*
Food Poisoning	*Wounds*
Gallstones	

Summary of Biological Activity

According to George Duke of the USDA, Turmeric has hundreds of molecular consituents, each with a variety of biological activites. On the following page we have included a table which lists these biological activites and the number of molecular constiuents of Turmeric known to have that activity. For instance, there are 20 constituents of Turmeric that are known to be bactericidal, (able to kill bacteria). Including these 114 activities, I counted 326 unique biological activities in his report. This is the power of using a whole herb over a single molecule. The healing picture of an herb is vast, especially when compared to a simple drug.

Biological Activity and Number of Constituents in Turmeric having this activity: George Duke, USDA

Bactericide	20	Antidiabetic	06
Insectifuge	16	Analgesic	06
Cancer-Preventive	14	Immunostimulant	05
Fungicide	12	Hypotensive	05
Antitumor	12	Febrifuge	05
Antiinflammatory	12	Antiherpetic	05
Flavor	11	Antihepatotoxic	05
Antioxidant	10	Allelopathic	02
Allergenic	10	Antiasthmatic	05
Spasmolytic	09	Antiallergic	05
Perfumery	09	Phagocytotic	04
Herbicide	09	Lipoxygenase-Inhibitor	04
Choleretic	09	Irritant	04
Antiseptic	09	Insecticide	04
Sedative	08	Hepatoprotective	04
Antiulcer	08	Cholagogue	04
Nematicide	07	Antiperoxidant	04
Antiviral	07	Antiosteoporotic	04
Antimutagenic	07	Antiflu	04
Viricide	06	Antieczemic	04
Hypocholesterolemic	06	Antiarthritic	04
Expectorant	06	Anesthetic	04
Antiedemic	06	Ubiquiot	03
		Antialzheimeran	03
		Vulnerary	03
		Sunscreen	03
		Prostaglandigenic	03
		Motor-Depressant	03
		Laxative	03
		Hepatotonic	03
		Cytotoxic	03

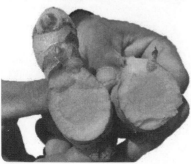

Antitussive	03
Antispasmodic	03
Antiradicular	03
Antimigraine	03
Antiinsomniac	03
Antifatigue	03
Antiepileptic	03
Antiencephalitic	03
Antidote (Lead)	03
Antidepressant	03
Antidecubitic	03
Anticataract	03
Anticariogenic	03
Anticancer	03
Antiatherosclerotic	03
Antialcoholic	03
Antiaggregant	03
Vermifuge	02
Termitifuge	02
RES-Activator	02
Mucogenic	02
Metal-Chelator	02
Immunosuppressant	02
Hypoglycemic	02
Diuretic	02
Dermatitigenic	02
Deodorant	02
Candidistat	02
Candidicide	02
Antistomatitic	02
Antiprostaglandin	02
Antiphotophobic	02
Antiperiodontitic	02

Anthelminthic	02
Antiphotophobic	02
Antiperiodontitic	02
Antipellagric	02
Antiparkinsonian	02
Antiosteoarthritic	02
Antiobesity	02
Antineuralgic	02
Antilepric	02
Antiischemic	02
Antiinfertility	02
AntiHIV	02
Antihistaminic	02
Antifeedant	02
Antidote (Cadmium)	02
Antidote (Aluminum)	02
Antidermatitic	02
AntiCrohn's	02
Anticonvulsant	02
Anticolitic	02
Anticold	02
Anticholinesterase	02
Anticheilitic	02
Antibronchitic	02
Antiarrhythmic	02
Antianorectic	02
Antianemic	02
Antiacne	02
Antipellargic	02
Androgenic	02

3

Turmeric in Ayurveda: Energetics

"The Earthy herb of the Sun." This reminds me of one of the Ayurvedic ways to see the inherent power of Turmeric, a power that is both balanced and which has a broad spectrum of action. According to Ayurveda, there are five great elements in the universe. These five mahabhutas, as they are called, can be loosely translated as Space, Air, Fire, Water, and Earth. Depending on which elements an herb manifests most, Ayurvedic herbalists can determine the action that it will have on the body. So let us look at Turmeric.

The Elements

It grows naturally in dark wet rich soil of the tropics. This means it must have a lot of earthy watery energy. This orange-yellow rhizome was also worshipped as an herb of the sun by the Vedic Solar dynasty of which Lord Ram was the pinnacle. This indicates that it must have solar or fire energy. Finally it has a strong bitter principle to it. The bitter taste has a cold air quality. The white-red-orange flower of turmeric makes the final connection to the etheric and so a case is readily made that it represents all five elements. This is a rare event in nature that signifies a broad range of power.

The Names

Every Ayurvedic herb typically has dozens of names that point to different aspects of the herb including its appearance, it's mythology, and it's healing ability. Today, the most common Sanskrit name for turmeric is Haridra. Some of its other Sanskrit names are Aushadi, Rajani, Gauri, Varnavati, Kanchani, and Nisha. Haridra can be translated to mean "the yellow One". However, the Vedic Rishis were geniuses and fun loving and loved to pack a lot of meaning into a single word, since everything was memorized and very little was written down. So the fact that Turmeric is such a beneficial herb for the heart and the name of the heart is Hrdya, very close to Haridra, makes me think the Rishis were playing. Rajani can be translated as meaning "that which colors". Gauri means "the one whose face is light and shining". Kanchani means the "Golden goddess". The Hindi name is Haldi, which means yellow, but is close to the Punjabi name 'Haldhar' meaning being strong enough to yoke a plow to your shoulders. If you know a Punjabi you won't be surprised by such a name. My Guru is from the Punjab where most people tend to be big and strong and attribute some of that vigor to Turmeric.

To me the most interesting name is Aushadi. Aushadi is typically used as a general term to describe any healing herb. However, it is often used in the Vedas, the ancient books of wisdom, which are at least 10,000 years old, to describe Turmeric. This makes me think that they considered Turmeric to be 'Thee Herb', the most outstanding herb, the one herb above all others.

Other names are as follows

Name	Literal meaning	Expanded meaning
Bhadra	Blessed, Auspicious, Friendly, Kind	Can be used daily to invoke deep wellness
Dirgharaga	The color which remains	Turmeric dye is fast. Make a big pot of Turmeric Tea and soak some clothes in it while you stir
Gandha Palashaka	With long and fragrant leaves	The leaves smell quite a bit like mango

Gauri	The fair colored one	It has a fair color and it gives beautiful skin
Gharshani	Whose color comes from rubbing	If you rub the rhizome on something the object will be colored
Haladi	Golden yellow	
Haridra	Golden yellow	
Harita	Golden Yellow	
Hridvilasini	Joyous	It grants overall health and thus joy
Jayanti	The victorious one	It defeats so many diseases
Jvarantika	The destroyer of fever	
Krimighni	The destroyer of pathogens	
Kringhna	The destroyer of pathagens	
Kshanada	Giving Pleasure also night blindness	Reduces night blindness; increases wellness and happiness
Mangalapradha	Auspicious	It grants good luck and good health
Mangalya	A Divine gift	It has so many uses that it must be a gift from the divine
Nisha	Night or Vision	Increases Night Vision and Has its own light source
Nishahva	Night or Vision	Increases Night Vision and Has its own light source
Pavitra	Sacred	Since it is a gift from the divine it is sacred
Pita	Yellow warming	
Pitika	Yellow warming	

Uma	Goddess of Transformation and Splendor	Herbs are considered to be close manifestations of the energy of the Goddess. Uma is one of the 3 or 4 most special aspects of the Goddess
Varna datri	Gives color	Gives color to complexion and can be used as a dye
Varvarnini	The Chosen one	Those who take turmeric are chosen to be Wed.
Vishaghni	Destroys poisons and toxins	Is a remarkable antidote
Mehaghni	Destroys urinary problems	Treats diabetes as Meha is Diabetes
Yoshita Priya	A woman's favorite herb	Because it grants beauty
Yuvati	The young woman	Because it is the goddess that grants youth

The Doshas

To further understand the Ayurvedic descriptions of Turmeric and its actions one needs to understand Ayurveda and the interpretation of all phenomena in terms of dosha.

Ayurveda is an ancient system of disease prevention, health care, and healing. Conservative estimates place the origins of Ayurveda in the Himalayan Mountains 5000 years ago. In fact, 3000 year old Ayurvedic texts that comprehensively include everything from advanced surgical techniques to herbalism, and from obstetrics to geriatrics are readily available. This makes Ayurveda the most enduring time-tested and proven healing modality available in the world today.

In Ayurveda the diagnosis of disease and individual constitutions is in terms of three psycho-physical doshas, or humors, called Vata, Pitta, and Kapha. The literal meaning of dosha is 'fault' because these three humors are the three ways in which the body tends to move out of balance. Every person's psychophysical constitution can be described in terms of one or any combination of these doshas. The following is a short description of the three doshas.

The Vata dosha is symbolized by Air. Its principle is movement, transport and kinetic energy in the body-mind. Its Essence is Prana, the Life Force. Key words are light, cold, dry, fast, quick, changing, movement, and restlessness. When balanced a Vata person is energetic but quickly gets nervous and upset when the 'fault' is unbalanced.

The Pitta dosha is symbolized by Fire. Its principle is transformation, metabolism, and discrimination in the body-mind. Its Essence is Tejas, Inner Light and Radiance. Key words are hot, fiery, perceptive, and intense. When balanced a Pitta person is intelligent but can get angry and fiery when the 'fault' is unbalanced.

The Kapha dosha is symbolized by water. Its principle is integration, lubrication, potential energy and stability in the body-mind. Its Essence is Ojas, Primal Vitality. Key words are slow, steady, solid, heavy, accumulation, and regularity. When balanced a Kapha person is steady and strong but can slowly become overweight and dull when the 'fault' is unbalanced.

Another important Ayurvedic method of describing an herb is by its guna, or quality. There are three gunas: Sattva, Rajas, and Tamas. Sattvic is purity, balance, calm, and is the underlying nature of the mind. Sattva is the typical picture of a monk. Steamed fresh vegetables are sattvic. Rajas is activity, typified by the warrior. Creation and herbs like black pepper or chilies are Rajas. Tamas is inertia, the tendency to remain unmoving. Old processed food and the couch potato are examples of Tamas.

Energetics of Turmeric

Turmeric is pungent and bitter in taste, dry and light in quality, hot in potency and bitter as a post digestive. Because it is pungent and warming it pacifies Kapha and Vata. It is bitter and astringent and so it pacifies the Pitta dosha. In general it is considered tridoshic which means it is used to balance all three doshas. Turmeric is predominantly Sattvic but leans toward being Rajas, sort of like a combination of a playful monk with a job to do and a calm noble warrior.

Primary Use in Ayurveda

To purify the blood and remedy skin conditions is the most common use of Turmeric in Ayurveda. The principle organs that it treats are the skin, heart, liver and lungs.

In Ayurvedic terms the uses of Turmeric include the following:

Vedana sthapana: Acts on the nervous system. Because it is anti-vata it helps to remove pain, insanity, epilepsy, etc.

Sangrahani: Treats chronic malabsorption

Anulomana: Purges out wastes (destroys worms, purifies blood, builds blood.

Rakta stambhaka: Stops excessive flow of blood

The list goes on and on and includes: appetizer, diuretic, purifies the uterus, purifies the milk, purifies and builds the semen, reduces fevers in the body, diarrhea, urinary disorders, insanity, poisoning, cough, and lactation problems in general. Sushruta, considered the "Father of modern surgery," recommended it for epilepsy and bleeding disorders. Charaka, who compiled a book on Ayurveda about 3000 years ago, recommends it for skin diseases and to purify the bodymind, and to help the lungs expel phlegm. It is used to treat external ulcers that respond to nothing else. Turmeric decreases Kapha and so is used to remove mucus in the throat, watery discharges like leucorrhea, and any pus in the eyes, ears, or in wounds, etc.

4

Turmeric in History

"I have found a plant that has all the qualities of Saffron, but it is a root."

Marco Polo on Turmeric, 1280 AD

The use of Turmeric goes back as far as we can see into History. Since it grows in South India, home of the ancient Dravidian race, and is a fairly obvious plant with so many potential uses, it is easy to postulate that it has been used for tens of thousands of years.

It was used to worship the Sun during the Solar period of India, a time when Lord Rama walked the Earth around 10,000 years ago. Perhaps it is because of its golden color that it is used in the worship of the sun even today. Especially in South India, you can see people wearing around their neck a hard dried turmeric root bead the size of a large grape. It is worn this way as a talisman to ward off evil and grant to the wearer healing and protection.

Every Brahmin male in India wears a Yagyopavita, a ritual sacred thread over their shoulder. Traditionally this thread is covered with Turmeric as part of the purification process.

As far as documented evidence, it is used daily in India for at least 6000 years as a medicine, beauty aid, cooking spice, and a dye. Women use it to lighten and perfect their complexion which would explain the name

"Gauri" which means "the light one". I would aver to say that this has been going on slightly less than 'forever'.

Buddhist monks have used Turmeric as a dye for their robes for at least 2000 years. It was listed in Assyrian herbal circa 600 BC and has been used at least for 1000 years in Chinese medicine. Curcuma was also mentioned by Dioscorides. In 1280 Marco Polo mentioned turmeric in his diary: "I have found a plant that has all the qualities of Saffron, but it is a root". So Europe has used turmeric as a substitute for saffron for at least 700 years.

One of the main active ingredients in Turmeric is Curcumin. This molecule was isolated by western chemists in 1815, obtained in crystalline form in 1870 by Daube, and its structure was determined in 1910 by Lampe. Turmeric has been used as medicine in the United States for about 30 years. Seems like the land where pushing frontiers is a way of life is understandably a little behind on this one.

5

Turmeric in Ethnomedicine

Turmeric in Chinese Medicine

As mentioned above, Turmeric has been used in China as medicine for at least 1000 years.

Yu Jin: Turmeric Tuber

In Chinese Medicine the tuber as well as the rhizome is used. The tuber, usually harvested in winter and spring, is called yu jin which can be translated to mean "constrained metal" or "constrained gold". It is considered acrid, bitter, and cool and enters the heart, lung and liver meridians where it stimulates blood and the movement of chi and thus breaks up stagnation. It is also used topically for pain relief, to reduce inflammation, and heal sores in skin, much the same way as it is used in Ayurveda.

Internally it is used when stagnant liver chi causes chest, stomach, side or menstrual pain and is good for the gall bladder and jaundice. It also clears heart and cools the blood and so is used when hot phlegm obstructs heart causing anxiety, agitation, seizures, and mental derangement. As you know, congested hearts and hot blood are very common symptoms of those living in any high pressure society.

It is combined with Dong qua for menstrual disharmonies and with Buplereum for liver, blood and menstrual problems directly related with liver dysfunction.

Turmeric tuber is contraindicated in Chinese medicine when there is a yin deficiency due to blood loss and it is used with caution during pregnancy.

Jiang Huang: Turmeric Rhizome

In Chinese Medicine the rhizome of Turmeric, which is usually harvested in winter when the sprouts have withered, is called jiang huang meaning 'ginger yellow',. It is considered to have acrid, bitter, and warm properties that work throughout the body and especially enter into the Spleen, Stomach, and Liver Meridians.

The rhizome has many uses based on its ability to stimulate and purify, and its actions as an anti-biotic, an anti-viral, and an analgesic. As such it is used to stimulate and strengthen the blood and decrease blood pressure, to clear abdominal pain and stagnation in men, women and children, and to remove stagnant chi, the pain due to stagnant chi, and excessive wind element. It is considered one of the better herbs for women because it stimulates the uterus and clears menstrual stagnation, dysmenorrhea and amenorrhea due to congested blood arising from a lack of heat or simply a deficiency. As in Ayurveda, it is a primary herb to treat pain and inflammation due to trauma. It is also used for wind dampness obstructions, especially in the shoulders, and to stimulate the gall bladder and normalize the composition of bile.

Turmeric rhizome combines well with cinnamon bark for menstrual problems and post partum pain due to blood stagnation; with cinnamon twigs and astragulus for cold induced blood stagnation, especially shoulder pain; and it combines with Dong qua for painful wind dampness obstructions. It also combines well with olive oil for topical applications.

Contraindications

It is sometimes contraindicated in cases of blood deficiency when there is no stagnant chi.

Dose

The dose of either the rhizome or tuber is typically 4 to 9 grams two to three times per day or 8 to 18 500 mg capsules per day. In terms of Curcumin, this could translate as two standardized 500 mg capsules three times per day.

Turmeric in Unani Medicine

"A root is a flower that disdains fame"

Kahlil Gibran

Unani is the name of the system of medicine that combines Ayurveda with the Greek Medicine encoded by people like Paracelsus and Hippocrates. Actually, Unani means Greek in the Persian language. The Unani tradition was a key link in the flow of medicinal knowledge from India to Greece. I have visited Unani Hakims all the way from the Nile to the Narmada because I am interested in their opinions and techniques. I appreciate the way they keep their herbs loose in drawers and give them to you in formulas spread out colorfully on sheets of white paper. Then they wrap each pile of herbs up in the paper and have you make a tea of them at home. It is a clear, clean, empowering interaction between you, the Hakim, and the herbs.

In Unani Medicine Turmeric is considered to be the safest herb of choice for all blood disorders since it purifies, stimulates, and builds blood.

You have heard of the phrase "Hot to the 3rd degree." I expect that the etymology of this phrase is with the Unani Hakims. "To the nth degree" is how they describe the potency of an herb, which can have any given quality to the 1st, 2nd, 3rd, or 4th degree. For Instance, Turmeric is considered hot to the 3rd degree and dry to the 3rd degree. Since Turmeric is often 10% oil, it is a little counter intuitive to say it is so dry or that its action is drying. Even the 'dry' powder is permeated with essential oil. Take a few ounces of Turmeric powder, put it in a standard plastic bag, and within a couple of days the oil will have penetrated through the plastic and the outside of the bag will be sticky.

Turmeric as Olena in Hawaii

When the ancient Polynesians made their fantastic voyages in canoes across the Pacific Ocean to Hawaii they took with them the roots, cuttings, and seeds of about 25 of their most valuable plants. Known as Olena, meaning yellow, Turmeric was one of these plants. To put this in perspective remember that this was a culture without iron or clay utensils and so plants were not just their food and medicine but also their tools, their containers and very much a part of their spiritual life. They were so much more in touch with the power of plants than we are today. Their tradition is carried on today by the Kahuna of Hawaii, the "Knowers of the Leaf". As in other cultures, they use Olena as food, medicine, dye, and for ceremonial purification.

As food and medicine the fresh juice or boiled root are used. The juice is extracted by pounding the fresh root and is used in earaches or to purify the sinuses via the nose. The root is also eaten to treat most pulmonary problems such as bronchitis or asthma. The Indian practice of applying the root paste to the face to cure any blemishes is popular in this tradition as well.

For ceremonial purification prayers are chanted as the mixture of fresh Olena juice and sea water is sprinkled on people, places and objects to remove negativity and restore harmony. For instance Olena is used in this way to cure someone who is very ill or to consecrate a newly built home.

Today in Hawaii, Olena rarely grows in the wild but it is organically cultivated by some who use techniques that are great for the Olena, great for the earth, and great for us.

6

Turmeric in Terms of Botany & Chemistry

The Latin name for Turmeric is Curcuma longa. It is a member of the Ginger family (Zingiberaceae). The Genus Curcuma contains about 35 species spread out throughout the tropical regions of the world. India has at least three of these species. The rhizome, which is the underground horizontal stem, is usually used. It is processed by first boiling, followed by curing, drying, grinding and extracting.

Appearance

Turmeric is a beautiful plant. When it comes up out of the ground it radiates it presence just beckoning to be noticed. It looks a lot like the ginger plant and the canna lily. The rhizome looks a lot like ginger before it is boiled. After it is boiled the whole rhizome turns yellow. The flowers, which blossom out of the center of the leaves, are white to yellow-red and bloom after the monsoon in the fall and winter. The leaves, which emit a sweet smell like the fruit and flower of the mango, are wide and deep green, pointed and oblong, growing out from a central stalk. They look like a short spear of a Zulu warrior. I use to live near a rural Ayurvedic Hospital in Oudh that grew all their own herbs. The Turmeric flowers stood out, even though they were next to the Hibiscus.

Preferred Climate

Turmeric is an earthy herb growing in hot, moist tropical climates where microbial attack would be standard. It has developed a chemical defense system from these attacks. It is this defense that also defends us from parasites, carcinogens, and oxidation when we use Turmeric. Botanists believe that it is probably indigenous to Bihar, the North Indian state famous for its Mithala art and Buddhist Holy places. Still today it grows there seemingly better than any other place in the world, with the possible exception of Orissa and Hawaii.

If you want to grow Turmeric, remember that it loves moist rich soil and shade. After planting the root will appear to be dormant for several months. Typically it is dormant during the winter months, and may appear to be dead as the leaves fall off, but the plant will come back with green leaves and flowers on a stem in the center of the leaf stalks. The yellow and white flowers clusters are several inches long and grow on the lower pale green. Turmeric is as visually attractive as it is medicinally healing.

On the Technical Side: Active Constituents

By far the most researched constituents in Turmeric are the 3 alkaloidal Curcumins which belong to the dicinnamoyl methane group: Curcumin, Demethoxy-curcumin, and Bisdemethoxy-curcumin. These are the gold substances in Turmeric. Most of the research done is with a 95% curcumin extract of Turmeric though Turmeric in its raw state is only 3-5% Curcuminoids. Root extract contains curcuminoids and bisabolene-type sesquiterpines such as turmerone, curcumene, and zingiberene. The root is 70% Carbohydrates, 7% protein, 4% minerals, and 4-14% essential oils which is mostly turmerone and atlantone and zingiberone. It also has vitamins, the oil turmerol, alkaloids, valepotriates, and is about 1% resin.

Curcuminoids are polyphenols and are crystallized from Turmeric oleoresin. They appear as a free-flowing yellow orange powder. Of the 3 to 5% curcuminoids in Turmeric, typically 85% is curcumin, 10% is Demethoxy-curcumin, and 5% is Bisdemethoxy-curcumin.

Turmerin, a water soluble antioxidant peptide from Turmeric, has been found to be an efficient antioxidant/DNA-protectant/antimutagen. Turmerin forms 0.1% of the dry weight of turmeric and is obtained in a crystalline form. It is a heat stable, noncyclic peptide containing 40 amino acid residues, and three residues of methionine, which are partly responsible for the antioxidant activity.

The fresh rhizomes have at least nine sesquiterpenoids including alpha-curcumene, arturmerone, xanthorrhizol, germacrone, beta-curcumene, beta-sesquiphellandrene, curzerenone, alpha-turmerone, and beta-turmerone. It also has at least one monoterpenoid, camphor. Four species of C. xanthorrhiza could be classified into two chemotypes by their bisabolane-type sesquiterpenoid compositions.

Other molecules in Turmeric are d-camphene, d-camphor, 1-a-curcumene, 1-ʙ-curcumene, turmerone, ar-turmerone, carvone, p-tolylmethylcarbinoldiferuloylmethane, turmerone, zingerene, phellandrene, cineole, sabinene, and borneol.

Synthetic Curcuminoids

As mentioned above, the natural curcuminoids are curcumin I (diferuloylmethane), curcumin II (feruloyl-p-hydroxycinnamoylmethane) and curcumin III (bis-(p-hydroxycinnamoyl)methane) and Curcumin IV.

Some of the synthetic curcuminoids are salicyl- and anisylcurcuminoids. Though I would recommend the natural curcuminoids over the synthetic any day, the man made curcuminoids are still very potent. . Salicylcurcuminoid may be the most potent anti-carcinogen among the synthetic curcuminoids.

7

The Aromatherapy of Turmeric

Of all the constituents of Turmeric it is most likely that the greatest heal-ing power is delivered by the essential oil and by the curcumins. The essen-tial oil is such a powerful part of the plant because it is a concentrated mix of potent and often rare and unique molecules. An amazing aspect of the molecules in an essential oil, which may number as many as 400-500 differ-ent species in a single oil from a single plant, is that many of them have re-ceptor sites in the neuro-endrocine system of the body. Furthermore, it has been postulated that some of the plant molecules with human receptor sites do not have a use to the plant itself. This would suggest an incredibly tight evolutionary bond between humans and herbs. The huge interest in society to return to the use of herbs, and to move away from modern western medi-cine, may be an example of the strength and depth of the bond that we have with herbs. This bond is so deep that the language of the Spirit is needed to be woven with the language of science in order to begin to describe it.

The essential oil contains hundreds of different medicines but the main ones are: Sesquiterpene alcohol 50%, Zingeriberene and other Sesquiter-pene hydrocarbons 30%, d-a-phellandrene 4%, cineol 3%, d-sabinene 2%, d-Borneol 2.5%, and valeric acid 0.1%. The essential oil taken internally or used externally it is anti-viral, anti-bacterial, anti-fungal, anti-parasitic, and anthelmintic (anti-worm). As with all essential oils care must be taken when using it internally. Internal dose of the oil is 5 drops in a glass of water or tea with a tablespoon of honey stirred in.

Some Turmeric essential oil is up to 65% Alpha-curcumene, a sesquiter-penic hydrocarbon. It is one of the main constituents of Turmeric respon-sible for lowering triglycerides and it has a high anti-inflammatory activity. It is found in the petroleum ether fraction.

The terpenoid Zingiberene and 6-gingerol are important digestive and carminative constituents. The essential oils contain Tolymethyl carbinol which is likely responsible for its liver support. Ar-Turmerone is used in tra-ditional Brazilian medicine as a potent anti-venom to neutralize the bleed-ing and lethalness of Pit Viper bites.

Case Study

Turmeric essential oil was given orally in a dose of 0.01 ml per kg and compared to 10 mg/kg of hydrocortisone. The Turmeric oils were found to be a better anti-inflammatory and anti-histamine.

The Ayurvedic Aromatherapy of Turmeric

Almost all oils, including Turmeric oil, decrease Vata because oil in gen-eral is the opposite of Vata. The sesquiterpene alcohols, which are detoxing and toning, tend to increase Pitta and decrease Kapha. However, sesquiter-penes, which are anti-allergy and anti-inflamatory, tend to decrease Pitta and so a balance is created.

8

Turmeric the Beautician

Health is the number one Beautician and Turmeric helps you to be healthy. But it does not stop at just granting the glow of a harmonious healthy bodymind. Turmeric cleans and purifies the blood and skin so that that glow of health is not attenuated by blemishes and impurities but rather amplified through clarity.

Secret Nature

As mentioned earlier, the Ayurvedic herbalist can predict an herb's actions on the body once the tastes and energetics of the herb are known. For instance, if an herb is bitter, you can predict that it will probably clean the blood and liver. About 90% of the actions of all herbs are predictable in this way. The other 10% tend to have unpredictable as well as uncanny powers. The unpredictable powers of an herb are called its Prabhava, which could be translated from the Sanskrit as its 'secret nature'. One example of this is the ability of sandalwood to transform downward rajas sexual energy into a more sattvic upward spiritual energy. Another example is Turmeric. The fact that it is so good for the skin is to some extent predictable, but the fact that it is incredibly great for the skin is due to a prabhava.

Vedic mythology often refers to herbs anthropormorphically, especially as gods, goddesses, and other great Beings who have incarnated as plants out of love and compassion for the planet. An example of this is Tulsi, Ocimum sanctum. So when I see the word Prabhava, which could also mean 'previous nature' I think that perhaps plants with Prabhava have brought that special power from a previous incarnation. This, of course, is all in terms of Vedic mythology, as mentioned. I would expect you could describe the same phenomena in terms of chemistry. I am musing now, but perhaps 'previous life' in terms of chemistry means that a plant which grew in the soil previous to the turmeric left special molecules which the Turmeric has taken and now delivers to you. My point is, though the languages and imagery of the ancient and modern can oppose each other 180 degrees, they may, in fact, be referring to the same thing, and thus neither need to be rejected by the other.

Skin

It is clear and simple: whether taken internally or applied externally, Turmeric is skin food. It both cleanses and nourishes the skin. It helps to retain the elasticity and youthfulness of skin. One of the reasons for this is that it is a cleanser that does not dry out the skin, but keeps it moist and lustrous. Turmeric is bactericidal and so can kill the bacteria that may otherwise cause your face and body to break out. It is traditionally used internally and externally to purify the skin and remove skin diseases like eczema and skin eruptions and even gonorrhea and open ulcers. Both ways will benefit the clarity and radiance of your skin. If you get a lot of sun or are exposed to a lot of pollution and smoke, turmeric will help protect you.

One way to use turmeric is to apply directly a thick paste made of turmeric and organic almond oil or sesame oil. Apply this cream directly on the inflamed area. The classic way to apply turmeric topically is as an Ubtan where you mix turmeric with chick-pea flour, oil as mentioned above, and a little fresh cream and honey. Turmeric is a great dye and will make your clothes and skin yellowish for a few days so take care when you are applying it. I permanently dyed my Champion yellow after juicing fresh Turmeric just once.

A good way to take it internally is to make a paste by boiling turmeric in water in a ration of 1:2. When it cools you can add maple syrup, honey, cinnamon, tahini, mustard, or whatever to make it taste better, then take a tablespoon of this paste at a time either straight, or in a sandwich, or in a glass of warm milk.

It is known that Turmeric, and especially Curcumin, inhibits skin cancer. It is likely that this action arises by decreasing the expression of proto-oncogenes. Once skin cancer has started Curcumin can also be used, again internally and externally.

External application stops swelling and heals wounds, stops pain, and stops skin diseases such from acne to leprosy.

Ubtans

Ubtans are mixtures of oils and herbs and grains that cleanse and rejuvenate the skin. A very simple classic ubtan is ghee and turmeric, which is known to make the complexion lustrous. In India this is done before weddings to make the couple very attractive. Another version is to mix wheat flour 4:1 with turmeric and add with honey and rose water to make a paste, and then rub your skin with this mixture. The advantage of this ubtan is that it does not make your skin yellow.

One of the many formulas for face and body packs is to simply mix turmeric with castor oil or coconut oil, smear the body, and then bathe.

Freckles

Freckles are known as Jhanyin in Sanskrit. I haven't figured out exactly why they happen in Ayurvedic terms but I am pretty sure that it has to do with Vata disorders in the Liver. Since Turmeric is a great Liver herb and is anti-Vata, taking it internally will help get to the root of the problem. Use the following freckle formula for a fine ubtan to treat them topically.

In the evening mix a large spoonful of Turmeric with Banyan or Bodhi tree milk until it is a uniform paste. Seal this in a jar overnight and massage it onto your freckles a half hour before your morning shower. Both the Banyan and the Bodhi tree are members of the Ficus family so if you can't find them it may be possible to substitute a more common milk producing Ficus in this formula. Remember that it will dye your skin yellow for a while.

Eczema

Since Turmeric is bitter and anti-inflammatory, it is excellent for hot skin diseases, especially eczema. According to Ayurveda, eczema comes from a hot liver, so another good remedy to heal this is to deal with any long term anger that may be stored in your liver. In this case mix turmeric with Gotu Kola to keep your mind as clear and happy as possible as you purify the liver with turmeric. Gotu Kola is also a wonderful wound healer, in fact it is one of the main herbs used to treat leprosy. So this combination would accelerate the healing of any wound, whether from a kitchen accident or a disease like leprosy.

Case History:

A woman in her late forties had very bad eczema since she was a teenager. It was so bad that she was often bleeding. Of course, she had tried everything. After two months on a very large dose of turmeric she beat the condition for the first time in 30 years and has had good skin since!

Since whole Turmeric is non-toxic and she was serious about getting rid of her painful condition the dose she was started on was approximately 30 gm of turmeric per day for several weeks.

Pox

In smallpox and chicken pox a layer of ubtan made from turmeric, fresh organic cream, wheat flour, and almond oil is spread on the skin morning and evening to increase healing and decrease scars. Doing this it still takes a month for the scars to heal. Raisin tea is also given internally.

Boils and Pustules

Not so many people in the West get boils or pustules but I have seen it happen many times to Westerners in India when their immune system starts to break down. They eat too many sweets, its about 120 degrees out for the 100th day in a row, and a minor staph infection goes systemic. By just taking a double or even triple dose of Turmeric capsules for a week or two, and cutting back on the gulab jamuns and other sweets, they find relief. Another traditional remedy for this is to take a pound of Turmeric and boil it in a gallon of water. Keep it covered so the essential oils do not escape. When it cools add a half pound of honey. Let this sit for two weeks. Boils are, of course, a very hot condition, and so to optimize the remedy it should be ruled by the moon. Thus, it is best to make the paste on the new moon and let it sit until the full moon. Then strain it and put it in a sterilized mason jar or glass bottle. Take a large spoon of it after every meal. If you don't want to wait two weeks, don't. Strain a quarter of the mix right away and start using that while the rest of it gathers strength and cooling power. Also apply Turmeric oil directly to the wounds. To make sure you do not tax your system any more than it already is, eat easily digestable cleansing food like soups and salads and stay away from dairy, sweets, bread and meat. Cooling herbal antibiotics like Neem and Goldenseal will also help.

If you get a fever by all means nurture it. It is one of the best therapies. I think it was Paracelsus who said. "Give me a fever and I will cure anything". So simmer between 101 and 102. If you get hotter, sponge bathe.

If you get cooler put on a wool hat, shirt, and socks. Fever releases the imbalance, the toxins, the pathogens. When you take action against a fever you are taking action against your body's inherent Wisdom, which is usually smarter than we are, and you end up driving the imbalance deeper into your body. Then it takes you a long time to slowly recover and you feel thick and groggy for weeks. On the other hand, if you go completely through the fever you soon feel so light and pure. As my teacher always says: "Your choice."

Scabies

Scabies is a contagious disease that results from a mite that burrows under the skin and then proceeds to drive you crazy. You end up itching yourself raw. Though most people will not get scabies, I have included it here to give yet another example of the power of Turmeric. I hope you never need to use Turmeric for this.

In the Ayurveda and Siddha system of medicine Neem and Turmeric have long been used for healing chronic ulcers and scabies. Again the Turmeric has many approaches to healing. As an anti-microbe it helps to kill the mites. As an anti-biotic, it helps to keep the wounds caused by the mites and the itching free of bacteria. As an anti-inflammatory it helps to control the itching. Finally, as a vulnerary, it helps to heal the wounds.

Case History:

In India a test was done with using Neem and Turmeric in a paste for the treatment of scabies in 814 people. In 97% of cases, cure was obtained within 3 to 15 days of treatment. No toxicity or adverse reaction was noticed in any of the subjects.

One old Ayurvedic doctor recommended that for scabies one should do a purgative of Turmeric and Amalaki, and then eat Turmeric and Neem, the whole while applying ghee and Turmeric externally. This he said will not only cure the scabies but leave the skin healthy. I would translate this into western context by recommending that for the purgative one take 5 to 10 grams of Triphala with 2 to 4 grams of Turmeric. Triphala is easier to find and is one third Amalaki. Then three times daily take 1 to 2 grams each of Turmeric and Neem internally. If the Neem is not available, substitute a cold antibiotic herb like Goldenseal. Finally apply ghee and Turmeric topically to the scabies or use sesame oil if the ghee is not available. This treatment can be used for most skin infections, ulcers, itch eruptions, eczema, ringworm, and skin parasites.

Tumors and Carbuncles

Fortunately, the word carbuncle is an obscure term for most people, but tumor still sends shudders through most of us. For an exposed tumor or carbuncle, take Turmeric rhizome and place it on coals. Reduce it to ash. If you store the ash place it in a glass jar with a good cover. Take the ash and form a paste with it with water. Take this paste and apply it to the tumor for 4 days 4 times per day. This will cause a wound in the tumor about an inch deep. Through this wound the tumor will pus and eventually die. After it has been reduced you can mix the ash with mustard oil and apply twice a day for two months. This will help with any ulcer that that does not respond to other treatments.

Leprosy

Fortunately, few people who read this book will ever need to know how to treat Leprosy, but if you do, apply a Turmeric tincture to the skin several times a day until there is relief. Simply take a wide mouth jar, fill it half full of Turmeric and the other half with vodka or brandy, and then leave it in the sun for one week. Normally tinctures are made in the dark for two weeks between new moon and full moon, but this tincture is to be ruled by the sun instead of the moon.

Shingles

For shingles take turmeric internally and also dust it over the shingles after applying mustard oil to the site of the infection. Traditionally they expect quick relief and a cure in 4-5 days. Turmeric flowers are traditionally also used in the poultice for shingles.

9

Turmeric as First Aid

Turmeric serves as First Aid in accidents ranging from cuts to concussions. For any trauma this rhizome is an herb of choice and is to Herbalism what Arnica is to Homeopathy or the Rescue Remedy is to Flower Essences. It helps to accelerate the healing of and minimize the damage from any trauma.

When an accident happens the body experiences stress and strain. If you can take the trauma out of your body before your body can memorize the state of stress you can significantly reduce the damage done and the time to full recovery. It is like running out into a blizzard in a T-shirt. If you are out for a few seconds you feel the cold but you do not get cold. In the same way, if you remove the stress from your bodymind as soon as possible, you won't be hurt as bad. Turmeric, Rescue remedy and Arnica help to remove the trauma out of your body before your body has a chance to memorize it. If you do not remove the trauma Ayurveda uses herbs, yoga and mantra to restore balance to both the body and mind.

Wounds

In India or in America, if I need to treat a cut I will pour 3% hydrogen peroxide on it first, if I have it, and then press turmeric powder into the cut or over the wound. I learned this from a chef in India. I was working next to her preparing a meal when I cut my finger quite badly. She put some curry powder in a small cup and had me press my bleeding finger into the powder. After a few seconds I took my finger out and the bleeding stopped. I left my finger covered with curry powder, which is predominantly turmeric, until the powder just naturally fell off, which was about 20 minutes. The wound never bled again and healed quickly. I couldn't believe how effective it was and am still amazed everytime I use this technique. There are so many more examples that I could give regarding the use of Turmeric in First Aid. Here is my favorite example:

Case History:

My teacher, Sri H.W.L. Poonja, was in a car accident in which a bone in his arm broke and came through his skin. Once the bone was set the surface wound remained open. After watching M.D.'s try to heal the wound for a week with allopathic creams I could not stand it any longer and used Vedic medicine on this Vedic Master. At his guidance, I made a paste that included Turmeric, Triphala, Neem, Honey, Rose Water, and an essential oil. This successful paste is a natural anti-biotic astringent vulnerary, and is useful to treat most open wounds.
As an anti-oxidant, you have to use Turmeric daily to be fully protected. However, in my experience in using Turmeric in first aid, I have found that it makes a significant difference in the healing of the wound even if you use it just once.

Road Rash

The main intercity transport in India these days is the scooter. Collisions with other scooters or with street pigs, falling into potholes, and getting blowouts are just a few of the ways that one can find themselves tumbling down the road, losing skin and getting a case of 'road rash'. To treat this I use the mix that I mentioned above to form an instant artificial scab that is antibiotic and healing. Spread the paste over the wound until it is about one eighth of an inch thick. If it is too thin it will not protect the wound and if it is too thick it will dry and crack and expose the wound. The natural scab would replace it in a few days.

Concussions/Contusions

I once was sitting in a micro-hospital in India with a dear friend, Swami Ramanananda Giri, waiting for a friend to be released. Though the friend had suffered some major blows to their body and head in an accident, we both felt that the iatrogenic blows were worse. The Swami was outraged and kept saying over and over:

In trauma we always give
in a tall glass of hot milk
two spoons each of Haldi and ghee.
This takes care of everything.

By reciting it like a Sanskrit sloka he permanently engraved it into my memory, though I am sure he was only venting his frustration and not trying to be didactic. Since then I have heard the same thing from many different sources. I have had the opportunity to test this since many traumas, from broken legs to broken hearts to drug ODs, and I am sure it works very well. By the way, ghee is clarified butter.

Sprains

Turmeric is known as a Yogi's herb because it helps to make the tendons and ligaments moist, flexible and strong. Having strong tendons will reduce the incidence of strains and sprains and if you are injured, Turmeric will help reduce the swelling, the pain, and will accelerate the healing. You can take large doses internally when you are injured as well as cover the affected area with turmeric. Blend the turmeric with almond oil and apply the paste to the sprain or wound.

Snakebites

One of the main constituents of Turmeric and Turmeric oil is ar-Turmerone. In traditional Brazilian medicine Tumerone is used as a potent anti-venom against snakebites to neutralized both the hemorrhaging from Bothrops jararaca venom, and the lethal effect of Crotalus durissus terrificus venom. Both of these snakes are genera of the Pit Viper family, known for their deadliness.

Insect and Scorpion Stings

As soon as possible apply a thick paste of Turmeric over the bite to antidote the poison, calm the inflammation, and heal the wound. You can also smudge the wound with Turmeric smoke to grant relief.

Scorpion bites are incredibly painful and can hurt for days. They can even prove fatal in some cases. Like the Cobra, scorpions come out in India during the monsoon because their hiding places are flooded. There is a Yantra, a powerful geometric design, that you can draw over Scorpion bites with a ball point pen which cures the sting in minutes. My Guru is so good at this yantra therapy that in Rishikesh, where there are a lot of scorpions, many people know him simply as 'Scorpion Baba'.

IO

Turmeric vs. Aids / HIV

When a virus replicates the 'long terminal repeat' (LTR) sequence is activated. Without this activation there can be no replication of a virus like the HIV. Published labrortory tests, completed by researchers at Harvard Medical School in 1993, indicated three inhibitors of HIV LTR. Curcumin is one of them and is shown to be effective against HIV in both acutely and, unlike AZT and most other anti-HIV drugs, against chronically infected cells.

Case Study:

Approximately 40% of the population in Trinadad are Indian and thus consume Turmeric in their diet on a daily basis. Another 40% of the population is African and rarely eat Turmeric. Africans in Trinadad are 10 times more likely to have AIDS than Indians in Trinadad. Of course, there may be many reasons for this huge difference, but it is quite likely that Turmeric is part of the reason.

On two proven accounts, Turmeric is definitely for anyone who is HIV positive or who wants to protect themselves from the human immunodeficiency virus:

*   *Curcumins have been shown to inhibit the replication of the virus.*
*   *Turmeric and the Curcumins have been shown to help the Immune system's T-cells survive and thrive.*

47

These facts are supported by tests performed both in-vivo and in-vitro. The Curcumins destroy the virus and keep it from replicating, and have a dozen or so healing side effects.

If I was HIV positive I would not rely solely on the Curcumins to protect me, but I would certainly use a lot of it in my treatment.

Case Study: In May 1993 a San Francisco man, infected with HIV, and who was having regular blood tests, starting taking 2 capsules of 300 mg of Curcumin in a turmeric base three times per day. After one week the tests showed a significant drop in p.24, which is a good measure of viral activity.

In India I use to always get shaved by the Barbers in the streets or down by the Rivers. You would just sit down next to them, they would lather you up, and shave you with a straight razor. It was almost a form of relaxing meditative body work, once you got over the fear of having a stranger hold a straight razor to your throat, and besides that, the shave was incredibly close. I stopped this practice many years ago when I heard reports about the spread of AIDS in India. Researchers had predicted that there would be a huge AIDS epidemic throughout India based on the following premesis;

* *There are tens of thousands of male and female prostitutes in Bombay alone.*
* *A large percentage of these prostitutes are "Vish", meaning poisonous, meaning carriers of the HIV, and a plethora of other STD's.*
* *There are millions of men who visit the prostitutes every year from all over the country.*
* *These men return to their homes and to local male and female prostitutes.*
* *Homosexuality is very common among Indian men due to social convention which makes it is so much easier for an unmarried Indian man to have a sexual relationship with one of his male friends than with a woman.*
* *I was being shaved by the same blade that shaved a hundred men a day.*

The bottomline to all this is that this epidemic, which had every right to happen, did not happen, at least not yet. Of course, there is a lot of AIDS in India, but not nearly what was expected. I expect that AIDS awareness is not a significant part of this. Rather, I would aver to say that exposed Indians are saved by Turmeric and other herbs and spices that they tend to consume in every meal.

For more information on Turmeric .vs. Aids please refer to the articles listed in the back of this book.

Turmeric for Immunity and Allergies

Your Immune system is very complex. When it is not working as fast as pathogens arise then you have a greater chance of getting sick. If it is able to keep up with the demands you are healthy. However, when it overworks, especially against a 'pathogen' that is not really harmful, you experience this as an allergy. Turmeric helps to normalize the Immune system by boosting it in times of need and calming it when it is working too hard for the given situation. In this way it displays an anti-allergenic effect.

II

Turmeric for Pain & Inflammation

Through Love all Pain becomes Medicine

Rumi

Turmeric as an anti-inflammatory herb is:

1. More potent than steroidal drugs
2. More potent than non-steroidals like indomethacin and phenylbuta-zone.

Therefore, it is very good treatment for:

- Arthritis and rheumatoid arthritis
- Injuries and trauma
- Stiffness from both under activity and over activity

Perhaps Turmeric's most important anti-inflammatory mechanism centers on its effects on the Prostaglandins.

Turmeric and Prostaglandins

Prostaglandins (PGs) are a large family of potent lipid biochemicals produced by the body. They are named after the prostate gland because they were first discovered in sperm and were assumed to be synthesized in the prostate. Their structure is similar to eicosaenoic fatty acids and are also similar to hormones because they stimulate target cells into action. But unlike hormones, which tend to act over the entire body, PGs act locally, near their site of synthesis, and they are metabolized very rapidly. Another unusual feature is that the same PGs act differently in different tissues.

Of the many different types of PGs the main ones we are interested in are PGE1, PGE2 and PGE3. PGE1 and PGE2 are anti-inflammatory, help keep blood platelets from sticking together, open up blood vessels, lower triglycerides, improve nerve regulation, enhance the functioning of T-cells in the immune system, and may help prevent cancer cell growth by regulating the rate of cell division. Flaxseed oil and cold water fish oil are foods that promote the production of these PGs. PGE1 protects cells and balances digestive secretions and so is useful in treating and preventing gastrointestinal mucosal diseases including gastric and duodenal ulcer disease, in inflammatory bowel disease, rheumatism, arthritis and other inflammatory disease. Together they are also the only effective therapy for preventing the total spectrum of induced mucosal damage from non-steroidal anti-inflammatory drugs.

PGE2 is inflammatory in nature, promote blood clotting, restrict blood vessels and increase salt retention. PGE2 can lead to water retention and high blood pressure, which are valuable functions under survival conditions, but under chronic stress, they are unhealthy. The body creates PGE2 from arachidonic acid, found mostly in animal foods, via enzymes called cyclooxygenase and lipoxygenase. This is one reason why consuming animal meat and dairy products increases your mental and physical tendency toward inflammation, aggression, and stress.

For millions of years our bodies evolved with an even ratio 1:1:1 of PGE1, PGE2, and PGE3, but now often experiences extreme imbalances of 1:45:1. This in part explains the increasing incidence of inflammatory disease and new problems like ADD in children.

Turmeric enters the PG and inflammation story because Curcumine is a potent inhibitor of cyclooxygenase, 5-lipoxygenase , and also 5-HETE production in neutrophils. Reducing these enzymes means less arachidonic acid metabolism, which means less PGE2, which means less pain and inflammation.

Arthritis

Traditionally, Turmeric is often used with Boswellic Acid (400mg 3x daily) as an anti-inflammatory to treat rheumatoid arthritis and osteoarthritis. Boswellic Acid is a constituent from the gum resin of Boswellia serrata. Turmeric is considered to be on par with cortisone as an anti-inflammatory, and some tests have found it to be 50% stronger. For joint pain, 1200 mg of curcumins have the same anti-arthritis activity as 300 mg of phenylbutazone. It protects the joints from inflammation thereby reducing arthritis. It blocks some of the pain and inflammation reactions and pathways and can deplete the neurotransmitters of pain. Another way that Curcumin works is by inhibiting the 12-lipoxygenase and cyclooxygenase activities in human platelets. The result is that it removes stiffness from whatever source: old age, arthritis, over exertion, or workouts.

Case History: Many athletes have found that taking turmeric reduces the pain and stiffness from a workout or event and shortens the recovery time.
In 1980 an Indian Hospital tested Turmeric on 49 rheumatoid arthritis patients. They were given 1200 mg of curcumin per day. Everyone of them improved in terms of less pain, more flexibility, and more energy.

Surgery

If used before and after any surgery it will decrease the pain and inflammation and accelerate the healing shortening the recovery time.

Yoga

Traditionally, yogis use Turmeric because it is so good for the tendons and ligaments. It helps them to attain and hold yogic postures and to avoid injuries. For more information see the section on Yoga near the end of this book.

Lime

Traditionally in Ayurveda herbs and formulas are often prescribed to be taken with lime. In this case mixing Turmeric with Lime is believed to improve its solubility and absorption. Modern analysis shows this mixture with lime gives rise to sodium curcuminate whose anti-inflammatory activity tend to be higher than that of curcumin.

Turmeric and Bromelain

For Pain and inflammation Turmeric combines well with Bromelain, which is extracted from the fruit and stem of the Pineapple plant. There are many studies as well as traditional wisdom that points to the strong anti-inflammatory activity of this extract. Bromelain contains proteolytic enzymes that split proteins into fragments such as peptones, etc, which is why it is also good for digestion. The dose of the Bromelain is 300 mg 4x/day.

Turmeric and MSM

MSM is Methylsulfonylmethane, a naturally occurring form of dietary sulfur. Sulfur, being an essential building block for many tissues in our body promotes healthy collagen, thus improving the form and function of skin, joints, tendons, and cartilage. MSM also increases the integrity of epithelial tissue found in your nasal passages, lungs, skin, and the lining of your digestive tract. It combines well with Turmeric in many cases including allergies, lung problems, any pain and inflammation, and parasites.

12

Turmeric, the Awesome Anti-Oxidant

The curcuminoids as an anti-oxidant compound are:

- 5-8x stronger than vitamin E
- 3x more powerful than Grape seed or Pine bark extract.
- More powerful antioxidants than Vitamin C, eugenol (from cloves), capsiacin (from cayenne) and BHT, a standard food preservative.
- Especially potent at scavenging the hydroxlyl radical, the most reactive of all oxidants.

This means Turmeric is good at:

- Keeping you feeling and looking young
- Protecting you from mutating cells, tumors, cancer.
- Preventing and removing oxidized cholesterol thereby preventing heart attacks.
- Reducing acute (injuries) and chronic inflammations (arthritis)
- Reducing pain associated with inflammation
- Preserving food

Anti-Aging

Everybody knows that oxygen is essential to life as we know it, but it can give rise to several reactive oxygen species (ROS) in normal metabolism. Normally the body can deal with these ROS but if there is an overload of them due to pollution, etc. or if there is an inability to deal with them due to genetics or weakness, then they can rapidly cause decay, breakdown, disease, rapid aging and death. Oxidation by free radicals can damage cells and DNA and thus is a major player in aging and a part to some extent of every chronic disease known. As rust is oxidized steel so aging is oxidized cells. Just as you wash the dirt and salt off your car to keep it from rusting, you surround your cells with anti-oxidants to wash away the oxidizing species of molecules. Proteins, lipids, and DNA are the parts of the cell most susceptible to damage by oxidation. Of course, oxygen isn't bad, it is the most needed nutrient to us, but reactive oxidizing molecules get out of hand. Actually one of the ways that our immune system destroys pathogens is to blast them with an oxidizer like Hydrogen Peroxide which rusts their little bodies within seconds. Most of the oxidants that we need protection from these days are a result of our modern day society: cigarettes, food additives, smog and pollution. Stopping oxidation stops a part of the aging process. Again, turmeric is considered to be the strongest antioxidant against the hydroxyl molecule, which is the most reactive of the oxidants. The phenolic nature of the Curcumins lend to Turmeric's anti-oxidant activity.

Prevention

Curcuminoids scavenge and neutralize free radicals and what is more amazing, they can prevent them from happening. One way that they do this is by blocking the oxidizing capabilities of metals. They protect the cells and chromosomes from cell damage.

Chronic Disease

Do you have a chronic disease or know someone who does? Oxidation by free radicals is linked with virtually every major chronic disease as well as with aging in general. There are many diseases directly associated with ROS production including: aging, atherosclerosis, cancer, cardiovascular disease, cataracts, hepatitis, inflammation, organic brain disease, rheumatoid arthritis, septic shock.

There are three ways to remove ROS. One is with anti-oxidants like Vitamin C and E and Curcumin. A second way is with certain enzymes which engage with the ROS and destroy its ability to react. Turmeric, a great anti-oxidant, has been shown to increase the number and activity of ROS destroying enzymes. The activities of superoxide dismutase, catalase and glutathione peroxidase in the liver are increased by turmeric. These studies indicate that dietary Turmeric lowers lipid peroxidation by enhancing the activities of antioxidant enzymes.

Food Preservation

Turmeric preserves food 3 times better than the common synthetic preservative BHT. This has been known for thousands of years in India, where refrigeration is only getting somewhat common in the cities since the early 1990's.

Daily Doses

Daily use of Turmeric is required to maximize its antioxidant properties. Experiments to study the mechanism of action of curcumin indicated that the presence of curcumin was essential for the inhibitory effect, as removal of curcumin resulted in restoration of cytochrome P450 activity and the levels of [3H]-B(a)P-DNA adducts to control values. For protection against anti-oxidants, it has to be there daily.

Not just the Curcumins

The curcuminoids, which are oil based, or lipophilic, and not dissolvable in water, are not the only anti-oxidants in Turmeric. This is evident since the water extract of Turmeric is also a strong anti-oxidant. Turmerin: a water soluble antioxidant peptide from turmeric has been found to be an efficient antioxidant, DNA-protectant, and antimutagen. Turmerin at 183 nM offers 80% protection to membranes and DNA against oxidative injury. ROS-induced arachidonate release and the mutagenic activity of t-butyl hydroperoxide are substantially inhibited by Turmerin. Tumerin is not toxic.

I3

Turmeric as an Anti-Microbial

Taken internally or used externally it is anti-viral, anti-bacterial, anti-fungal, anti-parasitic, and anthelmintic (anti-worm). The essential oil, the water extract, and the extracted curcumins all show this activity. You can use Turmeric to kill or inhibit microbes. It interferes with the ability of microbes and viruses to replicate themselves (see the information on Topoisomerase enzyme inhibition below) and it increases your Immune system to help with the fight against the infection. It is clearly proven to kill many bacteria in vivo and in vitro including staph and salmonella. Therefore it is great against staph infections and food poisoning. The fresh juice Turmeric is often used for many anti-biotic applications such as wounds or whenever an antiseptic is needed.

Case Study:

As an antibiotic Turmeric was compared with penicillin on gram positive organisms and with streptomycin on gram negative organisms. In both cases Turmeric came in second but gave a strong showing.
The side effects of penicillin and streptomycin include decreases in beneficial intestinal flora and immune system response. The side effects of Turmeric include beautiful skin, clean liver and blood, and increased immune system response.

Parasites

Turmeric protects you from parasites that can cause so many mental and physical problems, including poor digestion. People with intestinal parasite infections can get so mentally dark and contracted that I recommend joy along with Turmeric as part of my anti-parasite treatment. Though turmeric inhibits Entamoeba histolytica, Entamoeba coli and Giardia lamblia, I have used it more often to normalize the GI after treating an intestinal infection with other strong anti-parasites such as Kutaj, Clove, Black Cumin, and Cyperus. The alcoholic extract of turmeric is found to be anti-protozoal, especially against amoebas.

Aflatoxins

One of the threats to our health is aflatoxin, a very toxic substance pro-duced by Aspergillus molds which causes severe damage to the liver. These molds are most frequently found on peanuts and grains and occasionally herbs like black pepper. Turmeric destroys the mold and neutralizes the toxin and heals the liver. The curcumins also reverse the aflatoxin induced liver damage produced. Triple protection!

Case Study

A laboratory test was carried out to determine what substances showed anti aflatoxin activity. Turmeric, curcumin, asafoetida, butylated hydroxyanisole (BHA), butylated hydroxytoluene (BHT) and ellagic acid were found to inhibit the mutagenesis induced by aflatoxin. Turmeric and curcumin, which were the most active, inhibited mutation frequency by more than 80%. These results indicate the usefulness of Turmeric in ameliorating aflatoxin-induced cancer.

Anthelmintic

Traditionally, Turmeric is used to get rid of worms. One of its Sanskrit names, Krimighni, means "Worm Killer". It is interesting that the curcumi-noids are not anti-worm individually, but if given all together they become a potent anthelmintic. I always include Neem and Vaividong, Embelia ribes, in any anti-worm formula.

There is an interesting technique to get rid of worms and parasites that I am sure works. You bait them and then nuke them. First do a purga-tive and an enema to make room in your GI. For the purgative five to ten grams of Triphala will do as it is also antibiotic. Otherwise use Senna or Castor oil. You can also do the enema with Triphala tea. Then brew a very strong tea using one third herbal antibiotics, one third herbal carminatives, and one third herbal purgatives. While the tea is brewing eat sweets; chocolate will do. This, of course, is the bait. The pathogens will be overwhelmed with happiness and come out "in clear view", so to speak. In less than an hour their activity will make you feel a little nauseated and bloated. Then drop the bomb! Drink as much of the warm tea as you can, and I mean cup after cup. For relief from the tea, have a few cookies nearby to nibble on between glasses. Keep drinking lots of water. The idea is to kill or stun them enough so they can be easily flushed out of your system.

To be thorough, I then give anti-parasite capsules for a week, taking the nasty tea on the first, third, and last day of treatments. If you really want to be sure, wait a week and then do it again. If any cysts remained after the first attack you can get them with the second blitz after they hatch. Afterwards keep eating Turmeric and acidophilus, both of which will normalize your GI tract.

In this description I use pretty belligerent language. It is a sort of war, but one of your main weapons is happiness. Contemporary doctors will not believe this, but if you get mentally dark you get constricted in your body as well and this forms a knot in your GI that the pathogens will not be able to cross even if they wanted to. However, if you keep light and happy, even if it is fake lightness and happiness, you will open and allow the cleansing to happen. Believe me, it is true, I have seen this hundreds of times. I have seen one person cure her parasites with pure Joy and nothing else. With compassion, just send your parasites to a higher rebirth.

Anti-fungal

Turmeric is relatively broad spectrum anti fungal. One must remember that even though an herb is anti-fungal, it does not necessarily mean that it has a total spectrum or even broad spectrum of action on fungal infections. Each herb will have a different anti-fungal profile, and in fact, Turmeric has a different profile depending on whether you are using the oil or the extracted Curcumins.

Diarrhea and Dysentery

One of the main signs of a microbe infected is diarrhea and dysentery. Ten grams of turmeric in a cup of yogurt treats both diarrhea and dysentery.

14

Turmeric .vs. Cancer

And the winner is, in most cases, Turmeric. Of course it depends on how advanced the cancer is and on many other factors, but you have chosen well if you place Turmeric on your side in the fight against cancer.

Triple Action

Turmeric is considered to be anti- cancer because it has a triple action:

- It neutralizes those substances and conditions which can cause cancer
- It directly helps a cell retain its integrity if threatened by carcinogens
- If a tumor does grow curcumin can destroy the tumor

Triple protection

Turmeric definitely has anti-mutagenic, anti-tumor, and anti-carcino-genic properties. This means it neutralizes those things which can give you cancer. It helps a cell retain its integrity and not mutate into cancer. If a cell or cluster becomes mutated and cancerous, the curcumins can destroy the tumor. Triple protection from one herb. Turmeric fights carcinogens and cancer in every way and it can be used to both prevent and treat cancer, especially skin cancer, liver cancer, and colon cancer. In fact, Turmeric was recently nominated by the National Cancer Institute for study. One should at least use Turmeric as an adjunct therapy to standard allopathic techniques. Even if one was going the allopathic route to treat their cancer, they can still use turmeric to increase the effectiveness and decrease some of the side effects of cancer treatments. So many tests have shown that when the body is challenged by carcinogenic substances, Turmeric acts as an antagonist of many of these cancer causing agents and as a complete anti-dote to many of these toxins.

Ayurveda especially recommends Turmeric for cancers of the female reproductive system, namely breast and uterine cancer, and to treat benign tumors as well.

Topoisomerase Enzyme Inhibition

There are many reasons why Turmeric helps to destroy Cancer and parasites. One of the keys to this activity is the ability of the Curcumins to inhibit the Topoisomerase enzyme, which is required for the replication of cancer and parasite cells.

Topoisomerase site of action is within the nucleus of the cell, where it first binds to supercoiled DNA and then catalyzes the passage of one DNA helix through another via a transient double-stranded break. This splits the DNA and thus allows cell replication to occur. Since Topoisomerase , which contains 765 amino acids, is essential in cell proliferation, it is an ideal target in the treatment of cancer and parasites. Stop the replication and you stop the spread of the problem.

It is known that as parasites progress towards the stages where DNA replication occurs, there is a simultaneous increase in both Topoisomerase II production and activity. Also, cancer cells division requires this enzyme. In fact, if you can decrease this enzyme you even inhibit leukemia. Turmeric significantly reduces this enzyme. And since Topoisomerase is also one of the mechanisms that increases a pathogens resistance to drugs and the immune system, Turmeric is useful to minimize drug-resistant strains of pathogens.

Researchers at Michigan State University, found that Curcumin III (3) was the most active curcuminoid, inhibiting topoisomerase at 25 micrograms mL-1. Curcumin I (1) and curcumin II (2) inhibited topoisomerase at 50 micrograms mL-1.

Prevention

Once you have carcinogens in your system taking turmeric will help to neutralize them, but for optimal results it was found you should take turmeric before, during, and after exposure to toxins. Researched sponsored by the American Institute for Cancer research strongly suggests that Turmeric prevents and treats stomach, breast, colon, oral, and skin cancers. One reason for this is that Turmeric and Curcumins significantly reduce the level of DNA adducts when the cell is exposed to deadly carcinogens.

Dose

Prevention: 250 mg Curcumins 2x daily
Treatment: 500 mg Curcumins 3x daily

15

Curries & the Spice of Life

"Let your medicine be your food, and let your food be your medicine."

Advice from Ancient Greece

This is the dictum of the Greek 'Fathers' of Modern medicine. It is also a very basic principle in Ayurveda. In fact, there is a lot of evidence that the Greeks relied heavily on Ayurvedic Principles, techniques, and formulas as they came to Greece from India through Persian doctors like Avicenna.

To most people in India, from housewives to Himalyan hermits, Turmeric, affectionately called the kitchen queen, is the main spice of the kitchen, perhaps second only to salt in its ubiquity. In practically everything I have ever eaten in India, from Idli Sambar in a Tamil café to Jal Frezi in a Bombay 5 star hotel to rice and dahl with a Sadhu in a cave at 15,000 feet, Haldi is right there.

Turmeric adds a literal meaning to the phrase, 'The Spice of Life'. Curries are both a staple and delicacy of the Indian way of life for as long as there has been history, and Turmeric is the main spice in any curry which also typically includes ginger, cloves, chilies, black pepper, coriander, fenugreek and cumin. The standardized spice mix called curry is supposedly a British invention, as Indian cooking traditionally uses different proportions of the curry spices for every dish. Turmeric is also used to make pickles and mixed with ground mustard seed and vinegar to make 'Mustard'. Turmeric is absolutely essential in Indian cuisine.

Kitcheree

Basically Kitcheree is cooking rice and mung beans in Turmeric and a little ghee. There are as many variations of Kitcheree as there are cooks in India so there is room for experimentation around this central theme. Kitcheree is a simple meal served in practically every Ashram everyday, and in most homes two or three times a week. Kitcheree is famous for both its cleansing and nourishing action on the entire body. Usually cleansing and nourishing are opposite therapies in Ayurveda, but in the case of Kitcheree, and Triphala, both are possible at once, and hence it is one of the most recommended foods in Ayurveda. In fact, no description of turmeric would be complete without at least mentioning Kitcheree.

Digestion

Turmeric not only helps the food to be preserved outside of the body, but helps to digest it once it enters the body, especially proteins. Moreover, it heals and normalizes the GI. I use it during and after my anti-parasite cures to help normalize the GI after it had been totally upset with an amoebic infection. It helps to normalize the flora in the GI as well, especially the mucus membranes. Often GI parasites can cause colitis: little and not so little ulcers in the GI wall. Turmeric quickly patches up the holes and nukes the critters as well.

Food Preservation

Because Turmeric is such a strong anti-oxidant it inhibits the aging of food just as it inhibits the aging our bodymind when we eat the food with Turmeric. Turmeric preserves the freshness of the food, which is often important when there is a lack of refrigeration.

Certain amino acids can become carcinogens when heated to a high temperature. If turmeric is present it will inhibit this process and keep them nutritious instead of deadly.

Sakara Kaccha

In the traditional Brahman home there is a strong emphasis placed on purity. One of the manifestations of this is taking your food in the context of a ritual. Normal food is 'Nikara' and absolutely pure food is 'Sakara'. Sakara can only be taken in a clean room that has been sprinkled with ritual

water, usually from the Ganga. You can only enter this room if you have
just bathed and are wearing unsewn clothing, for instance a Dhoti or a Sari.
The purpose of such a ritual is to purify the bodymind with pure food and
environment. Now what makes this interesting for us is that in order for
the food, or Kaccha, to be considered Sakara, the great purifier Turmeric has
to be the primary spice.

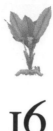

16

Turmeric & the Chakras

*There is a divine force that surrounds within and around a body
like a radiant sphere*

Paracelcus

Chakras mean different things to different people. In my experience,
they are energy transformers which transform zero point energy into manifest energy. Zero point energy is constant at any point in the Universe. It
is what the universe grows out of. If you take space-time and reduce it to
zero, at that tiny point is the gateway to infinite energy, zero point energy,
primal Shakti, Mahadevi. So the Chakra transforms that energy into the
great play of the energy, into what we know as our bodies and mind, into
swirls of consciousness. On the framework of the manifest energy the
mass which is us and the world precipitates like a cloud in thin air. So the
whole point of this paragraph is that golden turmeric is traditionally used
to cleanse and harmonize the Chakras and the channels of the subtle body
as well. Thus the energy of the Devi, of the Mother, is less directed by the
mental ruts which are our conditioned minds and more directed by a more
basic natural cosmic rhythm. This is not new age dreaming but a very basic
part of Ayurveda. As contemporary allopathic medicine takes you to be the
Newtonian machine of nuts and bolts, Traditional Medicine like Ayurveda
knows you to be pure energy, nothing but consciousness.

17

Detoxifying with Turmeric

Turmeric detoxifies the bodymind and in this way helps the body cure itself. One sure sign of this is that it increases the level of the enzyme glutathione S-transferase (GST), which is essential to detoxification. It also decreases obesity and you can be sure it does so in a very healthy way.

Turmeric is one of the dashemani, the 10 best herbs to treat poisoning and to purify. This is important because one of the Ayurvedic doctor's main jobs is to keep the King healthy and alive and one of the main ways that the king would become sick or die was by poisoning. Black Pepper Fruit is another one of these herbs.

Car Pollution

One of the main institutions in the World today is the car, or more specifically, the internal combustion engine. Though this device serves us very well in terms of transport, it is killing us in terms of pollution. Indian Cities are getting more polluted at an exponential rate. When I first came to India in 1987 there were not very many cars, but a lot of bicycles, rickshaws, scooters, and tongas, horse drawn carriages. Today the cars, trucks, and worst of all, the tempos, rule the road. Tempos are little 3 wheel mini buses which emit such a huge cloud of black exhaust that visibility in traffic can be cut at times to a hundred meters. Often I would go out on my scooter in a clean white kurta and come back in a gray one. In all this pollution the local people did not suffer as much as I thought they would. I believe that what is protecting them is the enormous amount of turmeric that is in their daily diet.

Case Study:

Laboratory animals were exposed to polycyclic aromatic hydrocarbons, car pollution, and tested for mutated cells in their urine, which is a standard method of determining how dangerous a substance is. Turmeric fed at 0.5% and above inhibited urinary mutagens, compared to controls. Turmeric did not adversely affect the food intake, or weight gain in the animals and no histological changes were detected. These findings are important in view of the widespread exposure of humans to polycyclic aromatic hydrocarbons.

Carcinogens

Besides car pollution and toxins, Turmeric helps to detoxify the body of carcinogens as well.

Turmeric has been found to be anti-cancer in-vivo and in-vitro in two respects. One is that is stops reactive processes from causing cancer. The second is that it detoxifies the body, not allowing toxins to accumulate and thereby decreasing the chance of a cell becoming a mutated.

18

Turmeric in your Ears, Eyes, Nose & Mouth

Teeth and Gums

I would aver to say that there is not an Ayurvedic toothpaste or powder that is worthwhile unless it includes turmeric. Due to its astringent, anti-biotic and anti-inflammatory properties, it is excellent for the teeth, in the form of a toothpaste, in your food, or just as a tooth powder to scrub on your teeth. In the latter case it is often combined with hot peppers and ash. It tones the gums and destroys bacteria whose acidic wastes cause cavities. And by the way, it does not turn your teeth yellow.

For toothaches or tooth decay, the standard remedy is Turmeric and Cloves. Either make a paste with water and apply it directly or tie a small amount of the dry powder in a small cloth and keep it next to the tooth until you have relief. You can also add Ajwain if you have it. Ajwain is one of these herbs that you either Love or you can't stand. Either way it doesn't matter as it will be dominated by the cloves.

For teeth burn turmeric into ash. Mix this ash with salt. Smear your teeth and gums with this for a tooth powder that will also treat cavities and gum disease.

If you ever burn your mouth swish and gargle with Turmeric tea.

Ears

Turmeric dust (with alum 1:20) is blown into the ear to treat chronic otorrhea.

Nose

You can mix a pinch of Turmeric with organic ghee (clarified butter) and apply it to the mucus lining of your nose to stop the sniffles. This also works for stopping nosebleeds and even helps to clear the sinuses and restore a more acute sense of smell. If you don't have ghee organic almond or sesame oil will also work.

In Ayurveda the brain is often treated with herbs taken via the nose because it is considered direct administration. There are many herb sensitive nerves that directly connect the nose to the brain. And so it is said that Turmeric applied in the nose helps to purify the mind and brain.

Eyes

One of the main causes of eye disease, especially cataracts, is the oxidation of lens in your eyes. Turmeric taken internally decreases the oxidation of the lens by causing a significant induction of glutathione-S-transferase isozyme rGST8-8 in the lens epithelium. That sentence may sound like Greek to you but it looks good to your eyes. It basically means that Turmeric helps to maintain the shape and integrity of your eyes.

Traditionally a Turmeric/water decoction (1 to 20) is used to treat conjunctivitis and eye disease in general. Soak a cloth in the decoction and then cover the eye with it. This helps to relieve the pain as well.

There is an eye-lotion called Mamira whose principle ingredient is Turmeric. Many elders in India attribute their great eyesight to the use of this traditional lotion. Unfortunately, most families have stopped using this home made compound. You won't believe how it is made. After placing two Turmeric rhizomes in a carved out hole in a Neem tree for about 6 weeks, take them out and grind them into a fine powder. Add a little camphor and rose water and you have Mamira. Apply it to the lower eyelid the same way eye shadow is applied. Folklore has it that this not only maintains visual acuity but can actually reverse certain types of blindness. Another version of this is to add Neem sprouts and the milk from a Bodhi tree. Grind this all together by hand for a week, each day adding new Bodhi tree milk. Legend is that this will make even the dullest eyes sparkle. It may be true, after all, the Bodhi tree is credited with granting Buddha his Vision of the Absolute Great Perfection.

I realize that most people reading this may never see a Bodhi or Neem tree, not to mention even a whole Turmeric rhizome. Yet I feel I must mention these things just to keep the Old Ways alive, and for that one person in a thousand who will actually do it.

19

Heart & Blood

As I write this book I can't quite figure out whether to address the action that Turmeric has on the blood in with the Heart, since the heart pumps the blood; in with the liver, since the liver cleans the blood; in with the skin, since clean blood means clean skin, or whether I should put all those under the one category of blood. All is interrelated and so Heart wins.

Blood Purifier

Turmeric creates new blood and so is good for anemia. It also purifies and moves the blood, which is one way that it is so good for the skin because it is hot, stagnant, and impure blood that predisposes the skin to blemishes and varicose veins. Curcumin is very similar to one of the active molecules in Chaparral, a great Native American blood purifier.

Hemostatic

It is a hemostatic, able to stop the bleeding of a wound. Most hemostatic herbs are bitter and astringent blood purifiers and so stop bleeding by cooling the blood and constricting the wound. Examples in Ayurveda are Neem, Manjishta, and Saffron. This is true of Turmeric but it is only part of the story. Turmeric also is a vulnerary, a great healer of wounds due to being both anti-inflammatory and anti-biotic. Since Turmeric is also pungent and warming it acts in the opposite way as well, breaking up platelets which are stuck together.

Blood Mover/Anti-coagulant

Traditionally Turmeric is used to move the blood, for instance in the uterus during the menstrual cycle. Also, there are platelets that flow in the blood whose job it is to form blood clots when we are wounded. The stress of being wounded causes the platelets to accumulate and stick together. In these days we experience a lot of the same stress without being wounded and our platelets start sticking together increasing the chance of a heart attack or stroke. Turmeric is known to inhibit this.

Cholesterol

Turmeric decreases cholesterol. Turmeric can stimulate the conversion of cholesterol to bile acids, an important pathway of elimination of cholesterol from the body.

Case Study:

In a 1992 study in India, 500 mg of Curcumin was given to ten people for seven days. After 7 days their total cholesterol count dropped an average of 27%. For many people that is the difference between the danger zone and death.

Heart Attacks and Stroke

Turmeric helps to prevent -strokes and heart attacks because, as mentioned above, it hinders blood clotting by reducing cholesterol and urging the blood to move more freely.

Turmeric for Diabetes

Turmeric lowers blood sugar. Therefore it is good for both diabetics and those of us who binge on sweets. Also, as it treats the liver and tissue, it will have an indirect effect on correcting diabetes.

Turmeric has been found to potentiate insulin activity more than threefold. Part of the action might be due to its chromium content. Turmeric likely also increases glucose metabolism.

Turmeric is an important herb in most Ayurvedic treatments of diabetes. Three times a day take a spoonful of Turmeric and honey paste mixed 1:4.

Also, eat bitter gourd fried with Turmeric and ghee as often as you can.

Turmeric the Diuretic

Turmeric heals urinary complaints, especially those that involve the Kapha dosha. There are three main Kapha dosha urinary complaints: sandra meha where the urine is dense and thick, pishta meha where the urine is colored like it is mixed with flour and smells bad, and shukra meha, where the urine is mixed with semen. Turmeric purifies all three of these conditions. Turmeric and Triphala are synergistic in treating urinary disorders.

20

Turmeric for your Liver

Turmeric is definitely one of the best herbs for the liver. I believe that Kutki (Picrorrhiza) is the best all around liver herb in Ayurveda, especially when it is harvested in Tibet. Ayurveda is actually full of great liver herbs and still Turmeric stands out as one of the best. A good liver remedy could be based on turmeric root, Kutki root, and Milk thistle seeds.

Turmeric removes cholesterol from the liver but also inhibits its assimilation, which means that it gives you double protection from cholesterol. Turmeric protects your liver from toxins and pathogens. It is known to both destroy major hepatoxins like aflatoxin and rebuild the liver after being attacked by hepatoxins. Turmeric also increases the secretion of bile, promotes bilification, and may prevent cholelithiasis.

If you drink more alcohol than your body can handle, you may want take a lot of turmeric to help your liver overcome the consequences of your habit.

Traditionally about 5 grams of Turmeric is taken with a glass of whey morning and evening to activate and rebuild a liver. This treatment usually lasts at least a month but it depends on the extent of the damage.

21

Turmeric for your Nerves

Traditionally, Turmeric decreases the air element in the body, which makes sense since it is a warming root from the still earth and air is cold and moving. Nervous energy follows very closely with the air element and so Turmeric soothes the nerves. Recent research proves Turmeric to be a very good antispasmodic.

Combine Turmeric with Ashwagandha and Brahmi to make an excellent nerve remedy. Even a disease as strong as MS will respond to these three herbs, especially if taken with high quality Omega 3, 6, and 9 oils as found in very fresh cold pressed Flaxseed, Borage, and Evening Primrose oils. This will calm the agitation and inflammation of the nerves and help to rebuild the myelin.

Turmeric is used traditionally in India to treat certain types of headache. It should combine well with Feverfew and Gingko in a headache formula, though I have never tried this.

Herbs are such a gift. They help cure us at so many levels. Religion really means Re-Ligio. Ligio is Latin and means 'to connect', like a ligament connects two bones. So re-ligio means to re-connect. Herbs reconnect us to the nature that we have extracted ourselves out of by becoming addicted to too much technology borne from a fearful mind. Eat a quick hamburger and you get in touch with a fast food chain and you reinforce the addiction and consequent separation. Eat or drink an herb from the mountain forest and you get in touch, reconnected, with a slow food chain, a chain that you have been evolving in for millions of years, a chain linked to every aspect of your being, a chain that your bodymind starves for. I guarantee this re-ligio, this reconnection, to be good for your frayed nerves.

22

Turmeric & the Respiratory System

After beauty and blood purification, support of the respiratory system is one of the main traditional uses of Turmeric in India. Mixed with the cooling digestives coriander and cumin it is excellent for calming a cough. With long pepper it becomes a lung tonic. As an anti-oxidant it protects the lung from pollution and toxins. It also helps the oxygen transfer from the lungs to the blood.

Asthma

Turmeric with ghee is traditionally used to get rid of cough and to treat asthma. If you feel that you are prone to an attack take 4-5 grams of Turmeric with a large glass of warm water. A more potent folk remedy involves roasting whole Turmeric rhizomes and mixing the ash with black pepper, rock salt, Bamboo leaves, and Babul resin.

Cigarettes

Curcuminoids have been shown to inhibit the mutagenic properties of cigarette smoke.

Case Study:

In 1992 at the National Institute of Nutrition in Hyderbad, India, anti-mutagenic effects of turmeric were assessed in 16 chronic smokers. It was observed that turmeric, given in doses of 1.5 g/day for 30 days, significantly reduced the urinary excretion of mutagens in smokers. In contrast, in six non-smokers, who served as control, there was no change in the urinary excretion of mutagens after 30 days. These results indicate that dietary turmeric is an effective anti-mutagen and it may be useful in chemoprevention.

Colds

Turmeric boiled in milk is used to treat coughs and colds and to decongest plugged up sinuses. Soon after I first came to India I was given a drink of turmeric and hot milk for a sore throat. It tasted very strong and it really helped. Turmeric is bitter, but unlike most bitter herbs, which are very cooling, Turmeric has a pungent side that adds warmth as well. As a pulmonary anti-biotic turmeric is a very good choice for bronchitis and other infections, especially when taken with fresh garlic.

Smoking Turmeric is traditionally used to destroy lung infections. Turmeric is burned and inhaled through the nose to get rid of colds and to calm hysterical fits! And it used to smudge scorpion stings.

For stuffed up noses try gargling with warm Turmeric tea for a minute and then blow your nose. Repeat this four or five times. It is best to do this between 6-10 AM and PM when the Kapha dosha predominates.

Pneumonia

Every treatment in Ayurveda is very specific to the person. The first thing to do is to check the state of the doshas and correct them. This will cure the root cause of the imbalance. But depending on the imbalance you may have to treat the symptoms first if they are threatening. Often Pneumonia falls in this category. One method to treat Pneumonia is with a Turmeric fomentation. The first thing to do is to get a rock or a brick and start heating it up in the oven or on a fire. Of course, don't make it too hot. If you do not have this a hot water bottle will do. While you are heating that make some strong Ginger/Black Pepper tea. Next, take a cloth and fold it several times. In the last fold put within the cloth a layer of Turmeric. Activate the fomentation by pouring the tea on the cloth. Place the cloth over the chest, again, making sure that it is not scalding. There should be one layer of cloth between the persons skin and the layer of turmeric. Then place the hot rock, brick, or water bottle over the cloth. There should be several layers of cloth at least between the hot object and the chest. Have the person sip the remainder of the tea.

Tuberculosis

Such a hard way to go. According to some Doctors in India, two grams of Turmeric, two or three times a day will restore the health in two months. If there is vomiting of blood, add the milk of a Bodhi or Banyan tree. In Ayurveda, there are many other therapies as well.

Hiccups

Did you know that a hiccup is "a sudden contraction of the diaphragm as air enters the lungs causing the glottis to close which produces an abrupt sound"? An Ayurvedic cure is to smoke Turmeric and urad dahl flour from a pipe. Take one long puff and see what happens.

Speaking of smoke throw some dried Turmeric on coals and inhale the smoke to quickly destroy mucous cough. In the same way you fumigate scorpion bites to grant relief.

I am really intrigued by Ayurvedic medicinal smoking of herbs. Except for the obvious, it is remarkable how underutilized this therapy is in the west. One of the uses of medicinal herbal smoke in the Ayurvedic and Native American tradition is to purify not just the body but also the psychic aspect of a person and an environment. So the smoke from these herbs actually is healing the room that you are smoking in as much as it is healing your body and your mind. Of course, this is the principle behind burning incense, smudge sticks, and even ear candles: Purify the subtle.

And speaking of therapies, some of the remedies mentioned in this book may be a bit hard to swallow in more ways than one and thus may paint a picture of Ayurveda as a series of obscure concoctions, all miraculously made out of Turmeric in one way or another. The truth is that Ayurveda has no peer in terms of the depth of healing offered. Furthermore, so many healing modalities have borrowed heavily from Ayurveda over the centuries including Allopathy, Unani, Tibetan, Chinese, Acupuncture, and Alchemy. A prime example is Sushruta, an Ayurvedic doctor who lived 2000 years ago, who is considered the Father of Surgery. He wrote a book on Surgery which is still studied by Western surgeons today. Another example is how medieval European alchemy borrowed from the discoveries of great eighth to tenth century Indian Saints such as Nagarjuna who practiced Ayurvedic alchemy to help their disciples attain Enlightenment.

Thyroid

I realize that the thyroid is not typically considered part of the respiratory system in Western Medicine, but in Ayurveda, it is a physical manifestation of the Vishuddhi, the throat Chakra, which governs the flow of the breath in many ways. It has been shown that taking standard doses of Turmeric resulted in statistically significant dose-related increases in the weight of the liver and the thyroid. These results were actually recorded at all dose levels.

23

Turmeric for your Stomach & Intestines

From one end to the other Turmeric treats the Gastro-Intestinal (GI) system. It increases bio-availability of the food that you eat and the ability of the stomach to withstand stomach acids. It nurtures mucus membranes and is traditionally used for weak stomachs, poor digestion, flatulence, and dyspepsia. It helps to normalize metabolism, and helps to digest protein.

Carminative

Turmeric is a great Carminative, which means it is an herb that calms an upset digestive system by getting rid of gas and distention. These herbs also tend to increase absorption and nurture the intestinal flora. According to Ayurveda, plants that treat digestion are the most important herbs of all since digestion is the basis of health.

Just taking Turmeric in capsule will work fine to balance an upset digestion. The folk remedy is to take a small spoonful of Turmeric and stir it in a cup of yoghurt. Take this after lunch and not on an empty stomach.

Gastric Ulcers

Laboratory tests show that Turmeric has a strong protective effect against food and materials that are corrosive to the stomach and intestines. Turmeric reduces the intensity of cysteamine-induced duodenal ulcers. Turmeric extract not only significantly increases the gastric wall mucus, but also normalizes gastric juices.

A Balanced Treatment

A carminative can be heating, in which case it calms Kapha and Vata but can aggravate Pitta, or carminatives can be cooling and calm Pitta, but possibly aggravate Vata. Turmeric is an excellent carminative because though it leans toward the heating pungent side with respect to the GI, it is very balanced and does not aggravate any of the doshas if taken in normal amounts.

Hemorrhoids

Use Turmeric with Flaxseed oil to treat hemorrhoids by both ingestion and topical application. To stop rectal bleeding take a 2 or 3 tablespoons of Turmeric every half hour until the bleeding stops, usually in an hour. A traditional remedy for "piles" is to directly apply to them a mixture of mustard oil, turmeric, and onion juice.

24

Turmeric & the
Female Reproducive System

Turmeric regulates menses, decreases intensity and pain of periods, decreases amenorrhea and decreases uterine tumors. Basically, it gets the uterus moving and back on a steady rhythm. Though I have not seen any technical paper on Turmeric's effects on hormones, I feel that it helps to balance those hormones which when out of balance can cause breakouts and disharmonious periods. Turmeric is a mild and supportive uterine stimulant. It will also help to normalize menstruation as it removes stagnant blood. It is great to take when you are pregnant in that the child will be benefited and traditionally it is said that then the child will always have beautiful skin. However, since it is a mild uterine stimulant there is a chance of over stimulation of the uterus. So if you are pregnant and would like to use turmeric, please see a qualified practitioner who can judge if it is safe for you to take it. Generally, women with more earth and water in their constitutions will be able to take the turmeric more often than a woman who has the air element dominating.

Contraception

As beautiful as it is to have a Child, in every culture there are dozens of folklore contraceptives. Ayurveda is no exception and one such technique is to take 5 grams of Turmeric, about 10 capsules, everyday during your period. Ostensibly, this will prevent pregnancy during your next ovulation. This effect is likely due to the action that Turmeric has on Prostaglandins, as described in the section regarding inflammation.

Emmenagogue

Its property of being an emmenagogue is closely related to its ability to purify and move stagnant blood. This helps normalize menstruation and tone the uterus.

Peri-Natal

India has not lost touch with natural birthing techniques, unlike the west which is just experiencing a revival of this critical knowledge. There are so many birthing tricks alive and well in India, and Turmeric plays an important role among them. For instance, in the last two weeks of pregnancy take two to three grams per day, or four to six capsules, with warm organic milk. This old remedy is reputed to not only simplify the birth, but it increases the health of Mother and Child as well. Remember to not take it too early: only in the last 10 days to two weeks of pregnancy.

The Midwife must be one of the oldest and most important professions on the planet. If at all possible I recommend incorporating a midwife into your life during pregnancy, birth, and infancy. A good Midwife adds so much Love, so much confidence in the natural process of birth, and so many natural techniques to serve the needs of the Mother and Child, and Father I might add.

I have always been amazed by the midwifery tradition in India. They belong to the Dai caste, which is a Sudra, a low caste socially, so it is not something anybody is allowed to do. But what is interesting is that while the woman of this caste assist in births, the men of this caste tend the burning ghats where your body is burned after you leave it. So together they act like the gatekeepers to Life. The Dai woman brings you in from spirit by birthing and the Dai man sends you off into spirit by burning.

Leucororrhea

For Leucorrhea take 10 grams of Turmeric and boil it in two cups of water. When the tea is cold use it as a douche three to four times daily.

Cancer

Experiments indicate that turmeric extract and curcumin reduce the development of tumors in animal. The anti-cancer activity of the rhizomes of turmeric was evaluated in-vitro in laboratory animals using tissue culture methods and in vivo in mice using Dalton's lymphoma cells grown as ascites form. Turmeric extract was cytotoxic to lymphocytes and Dalton's lymphoma cells. Cytotoxic effect was found within 30 minutes. The active constituent was found to be 'curcumin'.

Case Study:

A 1997 study at Tufts University School of Medicine, Boston, tested Curcumin and genistein (from soy bean) for their effect on breast cancer. Both compounds when present at micromolar concentrations were found to be able to inhibit the growth of estrogen-positive human breast cancer cells which had been induced by pesticides. When curcumin and genistein were added together to the cancer cells, a synergistic effect resulting in a total inhibition of the cancer. This suggests that the combination of curcumin and genistein in the diet have the potential to reduce the proliferation of estrogen-positive cells. The researchers concluded that "Since it is difficult to remove pesticides completely from the environment or the diet and since both turmeric and soybeans are not toxic to humans, their inclusion in the diet in order to prevent hormone related cancers deserves consideration."

Children

The benefits of Turmeric are definitely passed through the breastmilk to benefit the child as it benefits the mother.

It is so upsetting to see your infant or toddler suffering from a cold. A safe folk remedy is to put a pinch of Turmeric in breastmilk and have the child drink this 4 or 5 times per day. You may need to use a dropper.

25

Turmeric & Yoga

Turmeric as Food for the Yogi and Yogini

As a yogi and Ayurvedic practitioner I am most interested in the use of herbs to help balance your bodymind in order to minimize anything that distracts awareness away from the Oneness of all Being. Though I am bound by an oath of the Dharma to help you, it is naturally what I want to do anyway.

As everyone desires abiding Peace and contentment, so there is a Yogi in all of us.

As is shown, Turmeric is one of the best herbs for everybody. It is also one of the best herbs for Yoga because:

- It is one of the most potent purifying herbs in Ayurveda, cleansing all the bodies including physical and subtle, from muscles to marmas.
- It is one of the safest herbs.
- Turmeric increases flexibility.
- It reduces pain and inflammation from workouts which means it
- Allows one to perfect their asanas,
- Stay in asanas longer
- Stay in asanas with greater ease. The source books of Yoga declare that the Asana should be easy and relaxed.
- Increases Prana and the flow of Prana.
- Finally, Turmeric purifies Prana.

26

Safety of Turmeric

Though large doses are not recommended in cases of painful gallstones, obstructive jaundice, acute bilious colic and extremely toxic liver disorders, this is one of the most researched and most commonly known and used herb on the planet. In all the thousands of years of study and use, no known toxicity has ever been established, or even hinted at for that matter. On the contrary it is safe to say that today at least 500 million Indians take turmeric two or three times daily, and have been for hundreds of years. The human equivalent of a half pound of turmeric was given to rats for a year with no adverse effects. Normal toxic levels of drugs are 5 to 10 times the prescribed dose, and many drugs are toxic at their prescribed dosage. Turmeric on the other hand, is totally safe. It is what I would call a 'desert island Herb'. If you could only have a few herbs, this would definitely be a good choice for one of them.

The only issue against Turmeric that I have ever heard of is that, since it is so healing, it can cause a healing crisis. Suppose you want to sweep up a very dusty floor in your house. You come in with a big broom, open the doors, and sweep everything out into the street. As you sweep a cloud of dust rises in the room, and though the room is getting clean very quickly, the air is very dusty and uncomfortable. That uncomfortableness, as your body is cleansed, is a healing crisis. This crisis usually is no problem unless you are very weak. And that is the only warning I have heard about Turmeric: If you are really sick with an extremely toxic liver or obstructive jaundice, Turmeric may act too fast for your system and the healing crisis may be more than you want to go through. One option is simply take a lower dose and nurture yourself a little more.

Gupta found that large doses of Curcumin may cause stomach ulcers in laboratory animals. This leads me to address the issue of the safety of the whole herb compared with the safety of consuming a particular constituent of it. Often where an herb has a particular strong molecule capable of a strong biological action, nature places another molecule in the same herb that balances or anti-dotes the negative side effects of single molecule, yet does not diminish it action. This is why so many medical drugs have harmful side effects: they are single molecules with no balancing agent. This is also why I do not recommend taking single extracted constituents from an herb. For instance with Turmeric I would recommend a capsule with 100 mg Curcumins in a base of 400 mg Turmeric, and perhaps some Ginger and Licorice for assimilation and balance.

According to one slightly obscure Ayurvedic source, excessive use may be harmful to the heart in some people but this is counteracted with lemon juice.

In Chinese Medicine it is sometimes contraindicated in cases of blood deficiency when there is no stagnant chi.

The National Cancer Institute tested the toxicity of turmeric by feeding mice 2gm/kg of turmeric per day for 2 years! To the average human that is 140 grams or well over a quarter pound of turmeric per day. But what they gave the mice was concentrated resin of turmeric with 85% Curcumin which is equivalent to about 4 pounds of Turmeric per day. The normal dose is closer to 1 or 2 grams per day, or 1/100th of what they gave the poor little mice. I think 4 pounds of anything everyday would make you sick after 2 years, but after all that Curcumin the mice were relatively fine and Turmeric was deemed OK.

And indeed it is.

Epilogue

Professor Chunekar, one of the greatest herbalists of the last century, was taking me for a walk in the forest near the Ganga in Rishikesh one day. I asked him about Turmeric, and he quoted the passage on Turmeric from the Bhavaprakash, the best Herbal of Ayurveda, and one that he is praised for translating into Hindi and English from the Sanskrit. In the moment of this writing I couldn't find the passage, which would likely have taken this place. Alternately something else emerged, more contemporary.

Using This Ally in Daily Life

Ethnos likely comes from the Indo-European word for 'us,' or 'the people,' as in, 'we, the people,' the 'we, the people' that are one, without otherness, that are unified. I like to think that 'we, the people' include all Beings. Pharma means a medicine, a charm or an enchantment. Akeia means a remedy, solution, or resolution. Logos means the 'the word,' as in the word of the Truth of science and its study; and Logos also means the primordial source and fundamental order of the Cosmos.

Ethnos Pharma Akeia Logos is that Healing which resolves the people to align in harmony with ultimate source. Ethnos Pharma Akeia Logos is the ultimate medicine of the people that is given by our Nature and her abundance. Ethnos Pharma Akeia Logos is Ethnopharmacology. I am an Ethnopharmacologist and one of my goals in life is to make sure everybody becomes One.

So let me get real technical here and describe a few ethnopharmacological medicines.

Fresh Turmeric Juice

Often in Ayurveda swarasa, the 'self essence,' a plant's juice, is the strongest medicine. So juicing fresh Turmeric is one of the best ways to receive Turmeric's Power. Juice that amount of the fresh root that fits into your palm. You can drink this straight but most people prefer juicing it with carrots, ginger, garlic, celery and greens. Unless you live in Orissa, Ann Arbor, Paia or Fairfax you might not find fresh Turmeric so be an Activist and go online and make a list of all the Organic Turmeric farms in Hawaii, the Caribbean and Central America or wherever you are and see if you can get your local store to order it.

Turmeric in Smoothies

Simply put a teaspoon to a tablespoon in your smoothy.

Turmeric in Everything

As an Ethnopharmacologist I know that for thousands of years billions of people have been putting Turmeric in each meal of the day, usually right at the beginning of the cooking process. Soups, Salad dressings, Sauces (like 'Mustard'), Stir Fries, Bread, etc, all can have their flavor and their ability to enhance your wellness enhanced by Turmeric.

Swarasa

Epilogues reveal the fates of the characters in a story: All you people who have now read this book, you are 'we the people,' and for the fate of all beings I ask us as the ethnos to learn and use and share all we can about that pharma that will align us with Logos, Swarasa, and have a ton of fun making Akeia from our incredibly precious Plant Allies.

May all Beings be Happy.

Prashanti de Jager

About the Author

After receiving an M.S. in Aerospace Engineering from the University of Michigan and being on a PhD track in Electrical Biophysics there, Prashanti de Jager moved to India in 1990 and has lived there 10 out of the last 20 years sitting at the feet of a many great Advaita Saints and Tibetan Lamas. He studies and practices various Vedic Sciences including Advaita, Yoga, Ayurveda, Vastu Shastra and Jyotisha. Pioneering Organics and Biodynamics in India he has co-founded the herb companies Ayurveda Organics, Om Organics and Organic India which won the award for the Most Socially Responsible Company in the entire Natural Products Industry as it supports over 200,000 people in India to live in sustainable organic biodynamic fair trade havens. He worked for several years on the board of the California Association of Ayurvedic Medicine and is presently on the editorial boards of 'Light on Ayurveda Journal' and the 'American Herbal Pharmacopoeia.' He has taught numerous courses from Yoga Teacher trainings in Europe, North America and India, to Ethnopharmacology classes at the Mayo Clinic and U Conn Med School, to Panch Karma at the Rishikesh College of Ayurveda and Ayurveda at the Vedic Vidya Institute. He has consulted and designed herbal products for many companies including Christy Turlington, watched the well-acclaimed books on Vedic topics that he authored be translated into 12 languages and has published dozens of articles and herb photographs in magazines like Yoga Times, Yoga Journal, LA Yoga, Light on Ayurveda. See www.prashantidejager.com for more information.

Selected References

Traditional

Nadkarni, K.M., Indian Materia Medica, Bombay Popular Prakashan, 1976
Tierra, Michael; Herbology, Lotus Press, Twin Lakes, WI 1992
Zysk, K., Medicine in the Veda, Motilal Benarsi Das, New Delhi 1996
Frawley, D., and Lad, V., The Yoga of Herbs, Lotus Press, Sante Fe, 1986

General

Ammon HP, et al; Pharmacology of Curcuma longa. (Planta Med, 1991 Feb)
Anonymous; Clinical development plan: curcumin. (J Cell Biochem Suppl, 1996)
Aoi K, et al; [Studies on the cultivation of turmeric (Curcuma longa L.). I. Varietal differences in rhizome yield and curcuminoid content] (Eisei Shikenjo Hokoku, 1986)
Asakawa N, et al; [Determination of curcumin content of turmeric by high performance liquid chromatography (author's transl)] (Yakugaku Zasshi, 1981 Apr)
Bayat I, et al; Determination of selected trace elements in foodstuffs and biological materials by destructive neutron activation analysis. (Nutrition, 1995 Sep-Oct)
Chignell CF, et al; Spectral and photochemical properties of curcumin. (PhotochemPhotobiol, 1994 Mar)
Eaton EA, et al; Flavonoids, potent inhibitors of the human P-form phenolsulfotransferase.Potential role in drug metabolism and chemoprevention. (Drug Metab Dispos, 1996 Feb)
Francis FJ; Food colorants: anthocyanins. (Crit Rev Food Sci Nutr, 1989)
Futrell JM, et al; Spice allergy evaluated by results of patch tests. (Cutis, 1993 Nov)
Gewali MB, et al; Analysis of a thread used in the Kshara Sutra treatment in the Ayurvedic medicinal system. (J Ethnopharmacol, 1990 May)

Glaze LE; Collaborative study of a method for the extraction of light filth from ground turmeric. (J Assoc Off Anal Chem, 1975 May)

Goodpasture CE, et al; Effects of food seasonings on the cell cycle and chromosome morphology of mammalian cells in-vitro with special reference to turmeric. (Food Cosmet Toxicol, 1976 Jan)

Gorman AA, et al; Curcumin-derived transients: a pulsed laser and pulse radiolysis study. (Photochem Photobiol, 1994 Apr)

Goud VK, et al; Effect of turmeric on xenobiotic metabolising enzymes. (Plant Foods HumNutr, 1993 Jul)

Govindarajan VS; Turmeric--chemistry, technology, and quality. (Crit Rev Food Sci Nutr,1980)

Hasmeda M, et al; Inhibition of cyclic AMP-dependent protein kinase by curcumin. (Phytochemistry, 1996 Jun)

Hentschel C, et al; [Curcuma xanthorrhiza (Java Turmeric) in clinical use] (Fortschr Med,1996 Sep 30)

Holder GM, et al; The metabolism and excretion of curcumin (1,7-bis-(4-hydroxy-3-methoxyphenyl)-1,6-heptadiene-3,5-dione) in the rat. (Xenobiotica,1978 Dec)

Inagawa H, et al; Homeostasis as regulated by activated macrophage. II. LPS of plant origin other than wheat flour and their concomitant bacteria. (Chem Pharm Bull (Tokyo), 1992 Apr)

Kamikura M, et al; [Studies on intake of natural colors (I). Determination and presumptive intake of curcumin] (Eisei Shikenjo Hokoku, 1983)

Kaul S, et al; Effect of retinol deficiency and curcumin or turmeric feeding on brain Na(+)-K+adenosine triphosphatase activity. (Mol Cell Biochem, 1994 Aug 31)

Kawashima H, et al; Inhibitory effects of alkyl gallate and its derivatives on fatty acid desaturation. (Biochim Biophys Acta, 1996 Jan 5)

Lysz TW, et al; Identification of 12(S)-hydroxyeicosatetraenoic acid in the young rat lens. (Curr Eye Res, 1991 Apr)

Mair JW Jr, et al; Curcumin method for spectrophotometric determination of boron extracted from radio frequency ashed animal tissues using 2-ethyl-1,3-hexanediol. (AnalChem, 1972 Oct)

Marero LM, et al; Changes in the tocopherol and unsaturated fatty acid constituents of spices after pasteurization with superheated steam. (J Nutr Sci Vitaminol (Tokyo), 1986 Feb)

McNeal JE; Qualitative tests for added coloring matter in meat products. (J Assoc Off Anal Chem, 1976 May)

Patacchini R, et al; Capsaicin-like activity of some natural pungent substances on peripheral endings of visceral primary afferents. (Naunyn Schmiedebergs Arch Pharmacol, 1990 Jul)

Pradeep KU, et al; Influence of spices on protein utilisation of winged bean (Psophocarpus tetragonolobus) and horsegram (Dolichos biflorus). (Plant Foods Hum Nutr, 1994 Oct)

Rácz I, et al; [Stability of some curcumin dyes in solution] (Acta Pharm Hung, 1973 Jan)

Rao TS, et al; Some aspects of pharmacological profile of sodium curcuminate.

(Indian JPhysiol Pharmacol, 1984 Jul-Sep)

Roth HJ, et al; [On the color reaction between boric acid and curcumin. II. On the constitution of rosocyanins and rubrocurcumins] (Arch Pharm Ber Dtsch Pharm Ges,1964 Nov)

Shakila RJ, et al; Inhibitory effect of spices on in vitro histamine production and histidinedecarboxylase activity of Morganella morganii and on the biogenic amine formation in mackerel stored at 30 degrees C. (Z Lebensm Unters Forsch, 1996 Jul)

Shirota S, et al; Tyrosinase inhibitors from crude drugs. (Biol Pharm Bull, 1994 Feb)

Singh UP, et al; Effect of a new fluorochrome on pre- and post-UV treatment of Taphrina maculans Butler. (Z Allg Mikrobiol, 1977)

Srivastava R; Inhibition of neutrophil response by curcumin. (Agents Actions, 1989 Nov,Abstract available)

Stockert JC, et al; Fluorescence of plastic embedded tissue sections after curcumin staining. (Stain Technol, 1989 Jul)

Stockert JC, et al; Fluorescence reaction of chromatin by curcumin. (Z Naturforsch [C],1989 Mar-Apr)

Stockert JC, et al; New fluorescence reactions in DNA cytochemistry. 1. Microscopic and spectroscopic studies on nonrigid fluorochromes. (Anal Quant Cytol Histol, 1990 Feb)

Tennesen HH, et al; Studies on curcumin and curcuminoids. IX: Investigation of the photobiological activity of curcumin using bacterial indicator systems. (J Pharm Sci, 1987May)

Tennesen HH, et al; Studies on curcumin and curcuminoids. VI. Kinetics of curcumin degradation in aqueous solution. (Z Lebensm Unters Forsch, 1985 May,)

Tennesen HH, et al; Studies on curcumin and curcuminoids. V. Photochemical stability of curcumin. (Z Lebensm Unters Forsch, 1986 Aug)

Uehara S, et al; [Terpenoids and curcuminoids of the rhizoma of Curcuma xanthorrhiza Roxb] (Yakugaku Zasshi, 1992 Nov)

Wahlström B, et al; A study on the fate of curcumin in the rat. (Acta Pharmacol Toxicol (Copenh), 1978 Aug)

Wu H, et al; [Growth regularities of yujin (Curcuma longa L.)] (Chung Kuo Chung Yao TsaChih, 1992 Jul)

Yokoo T, et al; Dual regulation of IL-1 beta-mediated matrix metalloproteinase-9 expression in mesangial cells by NF-kappa B and AP-1. (Am J Physiol, 1996 Jan)

Yoshida M, et al; [Determination of boric acid in biological materials by curcuma paper] (Nippon Hoigaku Zasshi, 1989 Dec)

Yoshida M, et al; [Spectrophotometric determination of boric acid by the curcumin method] (Nippon Hoigaku Zasshi, 1989 Dec)

Yoshida M, et al; [Study on the histochemical staining of boric acid] (Nippon HoigakuZasshi, 1991 Dec)

Zhao DY, et al; [Separation and determination of curcuminoids in Curcuma longa L. and its preparation by HPLC] (Yao Hsueh Hsueh Pao, 1986 May)

Reddy, Vinodini, Krishnaswamy, K., Symposium on Therapeutic Potentials of Turmeric/Curcumin. Oct 1993

Aids/HIV

Burke TR Jr, et al; Hydroxylated aromatic inhibitors of HIV-1 integrase. (J Med Chem,1995 Oct 13)

Jiang MC, et al; Inhibition of HIV-1 Tat-mediated transactivation by quinacrine and chloroquine. (Biochem Biophys Res Commun, 1996 Sep 4)

Jordan WC, et al; Curcumin--a natural herb with anti-HIV activity [letter] (J Natl MedAssoc, 1996 Jun)

Li CJ, et al; Three inhibitors of type 1 human immunodeficiency virus long terminalrepeat-directed gene expression and virus replication. (Proc Natl Acad Sci U S A, 1993Mar 1)

Mazumder A, et al; Antiretroviral agents as inhibitors of both human immunodeficiency virustype 1 integrase and protease. (J Med Chem, 1996 Jun 21)

Mazumder A, et al; Effects of tyrphostins, protein kinase inhibitors, on humanimmunodeficiency virus type 1 integrase. (Biochemistry, 1995 Nov 21)

Mazumder A, et al; Inhibition of human immunodeficiency virus type-1 integrase by curcumin.(Biochem Pharmacol, 1995 Apr 18)

Sui Z, et al; Inhibition of the HIV-1 and HIV-2 proteases by curcumin and curcumin boroncomplexes. (Bioorg Med Chem, 1993 Dec)

Aflatoxins

Aziz NH, et al; Occurrence of aflatoxins and aflatoxin-producing moulds in fresh and processed meat in Egypt. (Food Addit Contam, 1991 May-Jun)

Firozi PF, et al; Action of curcumin on the cytochrome P450-system catalyzing the activation of aflatoxin B1. (Chem Biol Interact, 1996 Mar 8)

Soni KB, et al; Protective effect of food additives on aflatoxin-induced mutagenicity and hepatocarcinogenicity. (Cancer Lett, 1997 May 19)

Anti-biotic

Bhavani Shankar TN, et al; Effect of turmeric (Curcuma longa) fractions on the growth of some intestinal & pathogenic bacteria in vitro. (Indian J Exp Biol, 1979 Dec)

Dahl TA, et al; Photokilling of bacteria by the natural dye curcumin. (Arch Microbiol, 1989)

Anti-inflammatory

Ammon HP, et al; Mechanism of antiinflammatory actions of curcumine and boswellic acids. (J Ethnopharmacol, 1993 Mar)

Arora RB, et al; Anti-inflammatory studies on Curcuma longa (turmeric). (Indian J Med Res, 1971 Aug)

Chan MM, et al; Effects of three dietary phytochemicals from tea, rosemary and turmeric on inflammation-induced nitrite production. (Cancer Lett, 1995 Sep 4)

Huang HC, et al; Inhibitory effect of curcumin, an anti-inflammatory agent, on vascular smooth muscle cell proliferation. (Eur J Pharmacol, 1992 Oct 20)
Mukhopadhyay A, et al; Anti-inflammatory and irritant activities of curcumin analogues in rats. (Agents Actions, 1982 Oct)
Rao TS, et al; Anti-inflammatory activity of curcumin analogues. (Indian J Med Res, 1982Apr)
Reddy AC, et al; Studies on anti-inflammatory activity of spice principles and dietary n-3polyunsaturated fatty acids on carrageenan-induced inflammation in rats. (Ann Nutr Metab,1994)
Satoskar RR, et al; Evaluation of anti-inflammatory property of curcumin (diferuloyl methane) in patients with postoperative inflammation. (Int J Clin Pharmacol Ther Toxicol, 1986 Dec)
Srimal RC, et al; Pharmacology of diferuloyl methane (curcumin), a non-steroidal anti-inflammatory agent. (J Pharm Pharmacol, 1973 Jun)
Srivastava R, et al; Modification of certain inflammation-induced biochemical changes bycurcumin. (Indian J Med Res, 1985 Feb)

Antioxidant

Ashoori F, et al; Involvement of lipid peroxidation in necrosis of skin flaps and its suppression by ellagic acid. (Plast Reconstr Surg, 1994 Dec)
Awasthi S, et al; Curcumin protects against 4-hydroxy-2-trans-nonenal-induced cataractformation in rat lenses. (Am J Clin Nutr, 1996 Nov)
Donatus IA, et al; Cytotoxic and cytoprotective activities of curcumin. Effects onparacetamol-induced cytotoxicity, lipid peroxidation and glutathione depletion in rathepatocytes. (Biochem Pharmacol, 1990 Jun 15)
Huang MT, et al; Inhibitory effects of curcumin on in vitro lipoxygenase and cyclooxygenaseactivities in mouse epidermis. (Cancer Res, 1991 Feb 1)
Huang MT, et al; Inhibitory effects of curcumin on in vitro lipoxygenase and cyclooxygenase activities in mouse epidermis. (Cancer Res, 1991 Feb 1)
Joe B, et al; Role of capsaicin, curcumin and dietary n-3 fatty acids in lowering the generation of reactive oxygen species in rat peritoneal macrophages. (Biochim BiophysActa, 1994 Nov 10)
Krishnakantha TP, et al; Scavenging of superoxide anions by spice principles. (Indian J Biochem Biophys, 1993 Apr)
Kuo ML, et al; Curcumin, an antioxidant and anti-tumor promoter, induces apoptosis inhuman leukemia cells. (Biochim Biophys Acta, 1996 Nov 15)
Limasset B, et al; Effects of flavonoids on the release of reactive oxygen species by stimulated human neutrophils. Multivariate analysis of structure-activity relationships (SAR).(Biochem Pharmacol, 1993 Oct 5)
O'Donnell VB, et al; Role of oxidants in TNF-alpha-mediated cytotoxicity. (Biochem SocTrans, 1995 May)
Osawa T, et al; Antioxidative activity of tetrahydrocurcuminoids. (Biosci BiotechnolBiochem, 1995 Sep)

Rajakumar DV, et al; Antioxidant properties of dehydrozingerone and curcumin in rat brain homogenates. (Mol Cell Biochem, 1994 Nov 9)

Rajakumar DV, et al; Antioxidant properties of phenyl styryl ketones. (Free Radic Res,1995 Apr)

Reddy AC, et al; Studies on spice principles as antioxidants in the inhibition of lipid peroxidation of rat liver microsomes. (Mol Cell Biochem, 1992 Apr)

Reddy AC, et al; Studies on the inhibitory effects of curcumin and eugenol on the formation of reactive oxygen species and the oxidation of ferrous iron. (Mol Cell Biochem, 1994 Aug 17)

Reddy S, et al; Curcumin is a non-competitive and selective inhibitor of phosphorylase kinase. (FEBS Lett, 1994 Mar 14)

Reszka K, et al; Photosensitized generation of superoxide radical in aprotic solvents: an EPR and spin trapping study. (Free Radic Res Commun, 1993)

Sahu SC, et al; Effect of ascorbic acid and curcumin on quercetin-induced nuclear DNA damage, lipid peroxidation and protein degradation. (Cancer Lett, 1992 Apr 30, Abstractavailable)

Selvam R, et al; The anti-oxidant activity of turmeric (Curcuma longa). (J Ethnopharmacol,1995 Jul 7)

Shalini VK, et al; Lipid peroxide induced DNA damage: protection by turmeric (Curcumalonga). (Mol Cell Biochem, 1987 Sep)

Sharma OP; Antioxidant activity of curcumin and related compounds. (BiochemPharmacol, 1976 Aug 1)

Souchard JP, et al; [Substituted methoxyphenol with antioxidative activity: correlation between physicochemical and biological results] (C R Seances Soc Biol Fil, 1995,)

Sreejayan N, et al; Free radical scavenging activity of curcuminoids. (Arzneimittelforschung, 1996 Feb)

Sreejayan, et al; Curcuminoids as potent inhibitors of lipid peroxidation. (J Pharm-Pharmacol, 1994 Dec)

Sreejayan, et al; Nitric oxide scavenging by curcuminoids. (J Pharm Pharmacol, 1997 Jan)

Srinivas L, et al; Turmerin: a water soluble antioxidant peptide from turmeric [Curcuma longa](Arch Biochem Biophys, 1992 Feb 1)

Subramanian M, et al; Diminution of singlet oxygen-induced DNA damage by curcumin and related antioxidants. (Mutat Res, 1994 Dec 1)

Sugiyama Y, et al; Involvement of the beta-diketone moiety in the antioxidative mechanism oftetrahydrocurcumin. (Biochem Pharmacol, 1996 Aug 23)

Toda S, et al; Action of curcuminoids on the hemolysis and lipid peroxidation of mouse erythrocytes induced by hydrogen peroxide. (J Ethnopharmacol, 1988 May-Jun,)

Unnikrishnan MK, et al; Curcumin inhibits nitrite-induced methemoglobin formation. (FEBSLett, 1992 Apr 20)

Unnikrishnan MK, et al; Curcumin inhibits nitrogen dioxide induced oxidation of hemoglobin. (Mol Cell Biochem, 1995 May 10)

Unnikrishnan MK, et al; Inhibition of nitrite induced oxidation of hemoglobin by

curcuminoids. (Pharmazie, 1995 Jul)
Yokoo T, et al; Antioxidant PDTC induces stromelysin expression in mesangial cells via atyrosine kinase-AP-1 pathway. (Am J Physiol, 1996 May)
Zhao BL, et al; Scavenging effect of extracts of green tea and natural antioxidants on active oxygen radicals. (Cell Biophys, 1989 Apr)

Arthritis

Deodhar SD, et al; Preliminary study on antirheumatic activity of curcumin (diferuloylmethane). (Indian J Med Res, 1980 Apr)
Joe B, et al; Presence of an acidic glycoprotein in the serum of arthritic rats: modulation bycapsaicin and curcumin. (Mol Cell Biochem, 1997 Apr)

Aromatherapy

Apisariyakul A, et al; Antifungal activity of turmeric oil extracted from Curcuma longa(Zingiberaceae). (J Ethnopharmacol, 1995 Dec 15)
Hastak K, et al; Effect of turmeric oil and turmeric oleoresin on cytogenetic damage in patients suffering from oral submucous fibrosis. (Cancer Lett, 1997 Jun 24)
Salzer UJ; The analysis of essential oils and extracts (oleoresins) from seasonings--a critical review. (CRC Crit Rev Food Sci Nutr, 1977)
Tantaoui-Elaraki A, et al; Inhibition of growth and aflatoxin production in Aspergillus parasiticus by essential oils of selected plant materials. (J Environ Pathol Toxicol Oncol,1994)
Yasni S, et al; Identification of an active principle in essential oils and hexane-soluble fractions of Curcuma xanthorrhiza Roxb. showing triglyceride-lowering action in rats. (Food Chem Toxicol, 1994 Mar)

Cancer

Abraham S, et al; Mutagenic potential of the condiments, ginger and turmeric. (Cytologia (Tokyo), 1976 Sep)
Abraham SK, et al; Protective effects of chlorogenic acid, curcumin and beta-caroteneagainst gamma-radiation-induced in vivo chromosomal damage. (Mutat Res, 1993 Nov)
Ammon HP, et al; Curcumin: a potent inhibitor of leukotriene B4 formation in rat peritonealpolymorphonuclear neutrophils (PMNL) [letter] [published erratum appears in Planta Med1993 Feb;59(1):100] (Planta Med, 1992 Apr)
Anto RJ, et al; Antimutagenic and anticarcinogenic activity of natural and synthet-iccurcuminoids. (Mutat Res, 1996 Sep 13)
Aruna K, et al; Anticarcinogenic effects of some Indian plant products. (Food Chem Toxicol, 1992 Nov)
Aruna K, et al; Plant products as protective agents against cancer. (Indian J Exp Biol, 1990 Nov)

Azuine MA, et al; Adjuvant chemoprevention of experimental cancer: catechin and dietaryturmeric in forestomach and oral cancer models. (J Ethnopharmacol, 1994 Dec,)

Azuine MA, et al; Chemopreventive effect of turmeric against stomach and skin tumorsinduced by chemical carcinogens in Swiss mice. (Nutr Cancer, 1992)

Azuine MA, et al; Protective role of aqueous turmeric extract against mutagenicity of direct-acting carcinogens as well as benzo [alpha] pyrene-induced genotoxicity andcarcinogenicity. (J Cancer Res Clin Oncol, 1992)

Azuine MA, et al; Protective single/combined treatment with betel leaf and turmeric againstmethyl (acetoxymethyl) nitrosamine-induced hamster oral carcinogenesis. (Int J Cancer, 1992May 28)

Bhide SV, et al; Chemoprevention of mammary tumor virus-induced and chemical carcinogen-induced rodent mammary tumors by natural plant products. (Breast Cancer ResTreat, 1994)

Boone CW, et al; Screening for chemopreventive (anticarcinogenic) compounds in rodents.(Mutat Res, 1992 Jun)

Bouvier G, et al; Validation of two test systems for detecting tumor promoters and EBVinducers: comparative responses of several agents in DR-CAT Raji cells and in humangranulocytes. (Carcinogenesis, 1993 Aug)

Brouet I, et al; Curcumin, an anti-tumour promoter and anti-inflammatory agent, inhibits induction of nitric oxide synthase in activated macrophages. (Biochem Biophys Res Commun,1995 Jan 17)

Camoirano A, et al; Experimental databases on inhibition of the bacterial mutagenicity of4-nitroquinoline 1-oxide and cigarette smoke. (Mutat Res, 1994 Apr)

Chan MM; Inhibition of tumor necrosis factor by curcumin, a phytochemical. (BiochemPharmacol, 1995 May 26)

Chaudhary LR, et al; Regulation of interleukin-8 gene expression by interleukin-1beta,osteotropic hormones, and protein kinase inhibitors in normal human bone marrow stromalcells. (J Biol Chem, 1996 Jul 12)

Chen Y, et al; Transcriptional regulation by transforming growth factor beta of the expression of retinoic acid and retinoid X receptor genes in osteoblastic cells is mediated through AP-1.(J Biol Chem, 1996 Dec 6)

Chen YC, et al; Induction of HSP70 gene expression by modulation of Ca(+2) ion and cellular p53 protein by curcumin in colorectal carcinoma cells. (Mol Carcinog, 1996 Dec)

Commandeur JN, et al; Cytotoxicity and cytoprotective activities of natural compounds. Thecase of curcumin. (Xenobiotica, 1996 Jul)

Conney AH, et al; Inhibitory effect of curcumin and some related dietary compounds ontumor promotion and arachidonic acid metabolism in mouse skin. (Adv Enzyme Regul,1991)

De Flora S, et al; Structural basis of antimutagenicity of chemicals towards 4-nitroquinoline1-oxide in Salmonella typhimurium. (Mutagenesis, 1994 Jan)

Deshpande SS, et al; Effects of curcumin on the formation of benzo[alpha]pyrene derivedDNA adducts in vitro. (Cancer Lett, 1995 Sep 4)

Flynn DL, et al; Inhibition of 5-hydroxy-eicosatetraenoic acid (5-HETE) formation in intacthuman neutrophils by naturally-occurring diarylheptanoids: inhibitory activities ofcurcuminoids and yakuchinones. (Prostaglandins Leukot Med, 1986 Jun,)

Ghaisas SD, et al; In vitro studies on chemoprotective effect of Purnark againstbenzo(a)pyrene-induced chromosomal damage in human lymphocytes. (Cell Biol Int, 1994Jan)

Giri AK, et al; Sister chromatid exchange and chromosome aberrations induced by curcuminand tartrazine on mammalian cells in vivo. (Cytobios, 1990)

Han R; Highlight on the studies of anticancer drugs derived from plants in China. (Stem Cells(Dayt), 1994 Jan)

Han R; Recent progress in the study of anticancer drugs originating from plants andtraditional medicines in China. (Chin Med Sci J, 1994 Mar)

Hanazawa S, et al; Tumor necrosis factor-alpha induces expression of monocytechemoattractant JE via fos and jun genes in clonal osteoblastic MC3T3-E1 cells. (J BiolChem, 1993 May 5)

Huang MT, et al; Effects of curcumin, demethoxycurcumin, bisdemethoxycurcumin andtetrahydrocurcumin on 12-O-tetradecanoylphorbol-13-acet ate-induced tumor promotion.(Carcinogenesis, 1995 Oct)

Huang MT, et al; Inhibitory effect of curcumin, chlorogenic acid, caffeic acid, and ferulic acidon tumor promotion in mouse skin by 12-O-tetradecanoylphorbol-13-acetate. (Cancer Res,1988 Nov 1)

Huang MT, et al; Inhibitory effects of curcumin on tumor initiation by benzo[a] pyrene and7,12-dimethylbenz[a]anthracene. (Carcinogenesis, 1992 Nov)

Huang TS, et al; A labile hyperphosphorylated c-Fos protein is induced in mouse fibroblastcells treated with a combination of phorbol ester and anti-tumor promoter curcumin. (CancerLett, 1995 Sep 4)

Huang TS, et al; Suppression of c-Jun/AP-1 activation by an inhibitor of tumor promotion inmouse fibroblast cells. (Proc Natl Acad Sci U S A, 1991 Jun 15)

Jiang MC, et al; Curcumin induces apoptosis in immortalized NIH 3T3 and malignant cancercell lines. (Nutr Cancer, 1996)

Jiang TL, et al; Activity of camptothecin, harringtonin, cantharidin and curcumae in the humantumor stem cell assay. (Eur J Cancer Clin Oncol, 1983 Feb)

Kelloff GJ, et al; Chemopreventive drug development: perspectives and progress. (CancerEpidemiol Biomarkers Prev, 1994 Jan-Feb)

Kelloff GJ, et al; New agents for cancer chemoprevention. (J Cell Biochem Suppl, 1996)

Kelloff GJ, et al; Strategy and planning for chemopreventive drug development: clinical development plans II. (J Cell Biochem Suppl, 1996)

Krishnaswamy K, et al; Diet, nutrition & cancer--the Indian scenario. (Indian J Med Res,1995 Nov)

Krishnaswamy K; Indian functional foods: role in prevention of cancer. (Nutr Rev, 1996 Nov)

Kuttan R, et al; Potential anticancer activity of turmeric (Curcuma longa). (Cancer Lett,1985 Nov)

Kuttan R, et al; Turmeric and curcumin as topical agents in cancer therapy. (Tumori, 1987Feb 28)

Lin JK, et al; Inhibitory effect of curcumin on xanthine dehydrogenase/oxidase induced byphorbol-12-myristate-13-acetate in NIH3T3 cells. (Carcinogenesis, 1994 Aug,)

Liu JY, et al; Inhibitory effects of curcumin on protein kinase C activity induced by12-O-tetradecanoyl-phorbol-13-acetate in NIH 3T3 cells. (Carcinogenesis, 1993 May,Abstract available)

Liu Y, et al; Synergistic effects of curcumin on all-trans retinoic acid- and 1alpha,25-dihydroxyvitamin D3-induced differentiation in human promyelocytic leukemiaHL-60 cells. (Oncol Res, 1997)

Llorente AR, et al; Aluminium binding to chromatin DNA as revealed by formation of fluorescent complexes with 8-hydroxyquinoline and other ligands. (J Microsc, 1989 Aug)

Mukundan MA, et al; Effect of turmeric and curcumin on BP-DNA adducts.(Carcinogenesis, 1993 Mar)

Nagabhushan M, et al; Curcumin as an inhibitor of cancer. (J Am Coll Nutr, 1992 Apr)

Nagabhushan M, et al; Curcumins as inhibitors of nitrosation in vitro. (Mutat Res, 1988 Nov)

Nagabhushan M, et al; In vitro antimutagenicity of curcumin against environmental mutagens. (Food Chem Toxicol, 1987 Jul)

Nagabhushan M, et al; Nonmutagenicity of curcumin and its antimutagenic action versus chili and capsaicin. (Nutr Cancer, 1986)

Nakamura H, et al; The active part of the [6]-gingerol molecule in mutagenesis. (Mutat Res,1983 Nov)

Pásti G, et al; Curcumin does not alter the phorbol ester effect on cell-cell transfer of lucifer yellow CH. (Carcinogenesis, 1995 May)

Ren S, et al; Natural products and their derivatives as cancer chemopreventive agents. (ProgDrug Res, 1997)

Ruby AJ, et al; Anti-tumour and antioxidant activity of natural curcuminoids. (Cancer Lett,1995 Jul 20)

Sawai H, et al; Requirement of AP-1 for ceramide-induced apoptosis in human leukemiaHL-60 cells. (J Biol Chem, 1995 Nov 10)

Shalini VK, et al; Fuel smoke condensate induced DNA damage in human lymphocytes and protection by turmeric (Curcuma longa). (Mol Cell Biochem, 1990 Jun 1,)

Shih CA, et al; Inhibition of 8-hydroxydeoxyguanosine formation by curcumin in mouse fibroblast cells. (Carcinogenesis, 1993 Apr)

Sivaswamy SN, et al; Mutagenic activity of south Indian food items. (Indian J Exp Biol, 1991 Aug)

Smith WA, et al; Use of a microsome-mediated test system to assess efficacy and mechanisms of cancer chemopreventive agents. (Carcinogenesis, 1996 Jun,)

Sokoloski JA, et al; Induction of the differentiation of HL-60 promyelocytic leukemia cells by curcumin in combination with low levels of vitamin D3. (Oncol Res, 1997)

Soudamini KK, et al; Inhibition of chemical carcinogenesis by curcumin. (JEthnopharmacol, 1989 Nov)

Soudamini KK, et al; Mutagenicity and anti-mutagenicity of selected spices. (Indian J Physiol Pharmacol, 1995 Oct)

Stich HF, et al; The effect of retinoids, carotenoids and phenolics on chromosomal instability of bovine papilloma virus DNA-carrying cells. (Mutat Res, 1990 Aug)

Stoner GD, et al; Polyphenols as cancer chemopreventive agents. (J Cell Biochem Suppl,1995)

Takaba K, et al; Effects of n-tritriacontane-16,18-dione, curcumin, chlorphyllin,dihydroguaiaretic acid, tannic acid and phytic acid on the initiation stage in a rat multi-organ carcinogenesis model. (Cancer Lett, 1997 Feb 26)

Tanaka T, et al; Chemoprevention of 4-nitroquinoline 1-oxide-induced oral carcinogenesis by dietary curcumin and hesperidin: comparison with the protective effect of beta-carotene.(Cancer Res, 1994 Sep 1)

Thresiamma KC, et al; Protective effect of curcumin, ellagic acid and bixin on radiation induced toxicity. (Indian J Exp Biol, 1996 Sep)

Venkat JA, et al; Relative genotoxic activities of pesticides evaluated by a modified SOS microplate assay. (Environ Mol Mutagen, 1995)

Vijayalaxmi; Genetic effects of turmeric and curcumin in mice and rats. (Mutat Res, 1980Oct)

Yamamoto H; Interrelation of differentiation, proliferation and apoptosis in cancer cells. (JOsaka Dent Univ, 1995 Oct)

Cholesterol/Heart/Blood Lipids

Babu PS, et al; Hypolipidemic action of curcumin, the active principle of turmeric (Curcuma longa) in streptozotocin induced diabetic rats. (Mol Cell Biochem, 1997 Jan)

Dent RG; Defatting technique for two ground spices using simple reflux apparatus:collaborative study. (J Assoc Off Anal Chem, 1982 Sep)

Dikshit M, et al; Prevention of ischaemia-induced biochemical changes by curcumin &quinidine in the cat heart. (Indian J Med Res, 1995 Jan)

Hussain MS, et al; Biliary proteins from hepatic bile of rats fed curcumin or capsaicin inhibitcholesterol crystal nucleation in supersaturated model bile. (Indian J Biochem Biophys,1994 Oct)

Keshavarz K; The influence of turmeric and curcumin on cholesterol concentration of eggs and tissues. (Poult Sci, 1976 May)

Nirmala C, et al; Effect of curcumin on certain lysosomal hydrolases in isoproterenol-induced myocardial infarction in rats. (Biochem Pharmacol, 1996 Jan 12)

Nirmala C, et al; Protective role of curcumin against isoproterenol induced myocardialinfarction in rats. (Mol Cell Biochem, 1996 Jun 21)

Patil TN, et al; Hypocholesteremic effect of curcumin in induced hypercholesteremic rats.(Indian J Exp Biol, 1971 Apr)

Rao DS, et al; Effect of curcumin on serum and liver cholesterol levels in the rat. (J Nutr,1970 Nov)

Soni KB, et al; Effect of oral curcumin administration on serum peroxides and cholesterol levels in human volunteers. (Indian J Physiol Pharmacol, 1992 Oct)

Soudamini KK, et al; Inhibition of lipid peroxidation and cholesterol levels in mice by curcumin. (Indian J Physiol Pharmacol, 1992 Oct)

Srinivasan K, et al; The effect of spices on cholesterol 7 alpha-hydroxylase activity and on serum and hepatic cholesterol levels in the rat. (Int J Vitam Nutr Res, 1991,)

Srivastava KC, et al; Curcumin, a major component of food spice turmeric (Curcuma longa)inhibits aggregation and alters eicosanoid metabolism in human blood platelets.(Prostaglandins Leukot Essent Fatty Acids, 1995 Apr)

Srivastava KC; Extracts from two frequently consumed spices--cumin (Cuminum cyminum)and turmeric (Curcuma longa)--inhibit platelet aggregation and alter eicosanoid biosynthesis inhuman blood platelets. (Prostaglandins Leukot Essent Fatty Acids, 1989 Jul, Abstractavailable)

Srivastava R, et al; Anti-thrombotic effect of curcumin. (Thromb Res, 1985 Nov 1,)

Srivastava R, et al; Effect of curcumin on platelet aggregation and vascular prostacyclinsynthesis. (Arzneimittelforschung, 1986 Apr)

Xu YX, et al; Curcumin, a compound with anti-inflammatory and anti-oxidant properties, down-regulates chemokine expression in bone marrow stromal cells. (Exp Hematol, 1997May)

Detoxification

Susan M, et al; Induction of glutathione S-transferase activity by curcumin in mice. (Arzneimittelforschung, 1992 Jul)

Diabetes

Babu PS, et al; Influence of dietary curcumin and cholesterol on the progression ofexperimentally induced diabetes in albino rat. (Mol Cell Biochem, 1995 Nov 8)

Khan A, et al; Insulin potentiating factor and chromium content of selected foods and spices.(Biol Trace Elem Res, 1990 Mar)

Srinivasan M; Effect of curcumin on blood sugar as seen in a diabetic subject. (Indian J MedSci, 1972 Apr)

Ears

Rázga Z, et al; Effects of curcumin and nordihydroguaiaretic acid on mouse ear oedema induced by croton oil or dithranol. (Pharmazie, 1995 Feb)

Gastro-Intestinal Tract

Gupta B, et al; Mechanisms of curcumin induced gastric ulcer in rats. (Indian J Med Res,1980 May)

Huang MT, et al; Effect of dietary curcumin and ascorbyl palmitate onazoxymethanol-induced colonic epithelial cell proliferation and focal areas of dysplasia.(Cancer

Lett, 1992 Jun 15)

Huang MT, et al; Inhibitory effects of dietary curcumin on forestomach, duodenal, and coloncarcinogenesis in mice. (Cancer Res, 1994 Nov 15)

Ju HR, et al; Effects of dietary fats and curcumin on IgE-mediated degranulation of intestinal mast cells in brown Norway rats. (Biosci Biotechnol Biochem, 1996 Nov,)

Kositchaiwat C, et al; Curcuma longa Linn. in the treatment of gastric ulcer comparison to liquid antacid: a controlled clinical trial. (J Med Assoc Thai, 1993 Nov)

Pereira MA, et al; Effects of the phytochemicals, curcumin and quercetin, upon-azoxymethane-induced colon cancer and 7,12-dimethylbenz[a]an thracene-induced mammarycancer in rats. (Carcinogenesis, 1996 Jun)

Platel K, et al; Influence of dietary spices or their active principles on digestive enzymes of small intestinal mucosa in rats. (Int J Food Sci Nutr, 1996 Jan)

Rafatullah S, et al; Evaluation of turmeric (Curcuma longa) for gastric and duodenal antiulcer activity in rats. (J Ethnopharmacol, 1990 Apr)

Rao CV, et al; Chemoprevention of colon cancer by dietary curcumin. (Ann N Y Acad Sci, 1995 Sep 30)

Rao CV, et al; Chemoprevention of colon carcinogenesis by dietary curcumin, a naturally occurring plant phenolic compound. (Cancer Res, 1995 Jan 15)

Rao CV, et al; Inhibition by dietary curcumin of azoxymethane-induced ornithinedecarboxylase, tyrosine protein kinase, arachidonic acid metabolism and aberrant crypt fociformation in the rat colon. (Carcinogenesis, 1993 Nov)

Ravindranath V, et al; Absorption and tissue distribution of curcumin in rats. (Toxicology, 1980)

Ravindranath V, et al; In vitro studies on the intestinal absorption of curcumin in rats. (Toxicology, 1981)

Ravindranath V, et al; Metabolism of curcumin--studies with [3H]curcumin. (Toxicology, 1981-82)

Samaha HS, et al; Modulation of apoptosis by sulindac, curcumin,phenylethyl-3-methylcaffeate, and 6-phenylhexyl isothiocyanate: apoptotic index as a bio marker in colon cancer chemoprevention and promotion. (Cancer Res, 1997 Apr 1)

Wargovich MJ, et al; Aberrant crypts as a biomarker for colon cancer: evaluation of potential chemopreventive agents in the rat. (Cancer Epidemiol Biomarkers Prev, 1996May)

Wargovich MJ, et al; Inability of several mutagen-blocking agents to inhibit1,2-dimethylhydrazine-induced DNA-damaging activity in colonic epithelium. (Mutat Res, 1983 Jul)

Wargovich MJ, et al; Inhibition by plant phenols of benzo[a]pyrene-induced nuclearaberrations in mammalian intestinal cells: a rapid in vivo assessment method. (Food ChemToxicol, 1985 Jan)

Immune System/Allergies

Bosman B; Testing of lipoxygenase inhibitors, cyclooxygenase inhibitors, drugs withimmunomodulating properties and some reference antipsoriatic drugs in the modified mousetail test, an animal model of psoriasis. (Skin Pharmacol, 1994)
Douglas DE; 4,4'-Diacetyl curcumin--in-vitro histamine-blocking activity [letter] (J PharmPharmacol, 1993 Aug)
Kuramoto Y, et al; Effect of natural food colorings on immunoglobulin production in vitro byrat spleen lymphocytes. (Biosci Biotechnol Biochem, 1996 Oct)
South EH, et al; Dietary curcumin enhances antibody response in rats. (ImmunopharmacolImmunotoxicol, 1997 Feb)
Takeshita A, et al; TGF-beta induces expression of monocyte chemoattractant JE/monocytechemoattractant protein 1 via transcriptional factor AP-1 induced by protein kinase inosteoblastic cells. (J Immunol, 1995 Jul 1)
Watanabe A, et al; CD14-mediated signal pathway of Porphyromonas gingivalis lipopolysaccharide in human gingival fibroblasts. (Infect Immun, 1996 Nov,)

Liver

Baumann JC; [Effect of chelidonium, curcuma, absinth and Carduus marianus on the bile andpancreatic secretion in liver diseases] (Med Monatsschr, 1975 APR)
Fujiyama-Fujiwara Y, et al; Effects of sesamin and curcumin on delta 5-desaturation and chain elongation of polyunsaturated fatty acid metabolism in primary cultured rat hepatocytes. (JNutr Sci Vitaminol (Tokyo), 1992 Aug)
Hussain MS, et al; Effect on curcumin on cholesterol gall-stone induction in mice. (Indian JMed Res, 1992 Oct)
Jiang MC, et al; Differential regulation of p53, c-Myc, Bcl-2 and Bax protein expression during apoptosis induced by widely divergent stimuli in human hepatoblastoma cells.(Oncogene, 1996 Aug 1)
Kawashima H, et al; Inhibition of rat liver microsomal desaturases by curcumin and relatedcompounds. (Biosci Biotechnol Biochem, 1996 Jan)
Lahiri M, et al; Effect of four plant phenols, beta-carotene and alpha-tocopherol on3(H)benzopyrene-DNA interaction in vitro in the presence of rat and mouse liver postmitochondrial fraction. (Cancer Lett, 1993 Sep 15)
Lin SC, et al; Protective and therapeutic effects of Curcuma xanthorrhiza on hepatotoxin-induced liver damage. (Am J Chin Med, 1995)
Oetari S, et al; Effects of curcumin on cytochrome P450 and glutathione S-transferase activities in rat liver. (Biochem Pharmacol, 1996 Jan 12)
Panijel M; [Practical experiences in the treatment of gallbladder diseases] (Med Welt, 1982Jul 9)
Pilz R; [Therapeutic effect of Aristochol concentrate granulate in chronic cholecystopathies](Med Welt, 1975 Jul 25)
Reddy AC, et al; Effect of curcumin and eugenol on iron-induced hepatic toxicity in rats.(Toxicology, 1996 Jan 22)

Reddy AC, et al; Effect of dietary turmeric (Curcuma longa) on iron-induced lipid peroxidation in the rat liver. (Food Chem Toxicol, 1994 Mar)

Sambaiah K, et al; Influence of spices and spice principles on hepatic mixed function oxygenase system in rats. (Indian J Biochem Biophys, 1989 Aug)

Shah RG, et al; Evaluation of mutagenic activity of turmeric extract containing curcumin,before and after activation with mammalian cecal microbial extract of liver micro somal fraction, in the Ames Salmonella test. (Bull Environ Contam Toxicol, 1988 Mar)

Shimizu S, et al; Inhibitory effect of curcumin on fatty acid desaturation in Mortierella alpina1S-4 and rat liver microsomes. (Lipids, 1992 Jul)

Singh A, et al; Effect of arecoline on the curcumin-modulated hepatic biotransformationsystem enzymes in lactating mice and translactationally exposed F1 pups. (Nutr Cancer,1996)

Soni KB, et al; Reversal of aflatoxin induced liver damage by turmeric and curcumin. (CancerLett, 1992 Sep 30)

Yasni S, et al; Effects of Curcuma xanthorrhiza Roxb. and curcuminoids on the level of serum and liver lipids, serum apolipoprotein A-I and lipogenic enzymes in rats. (Food ChemToxicol, 1993 Mar)

Zhao ZS, et al; The prevention of CCl4-induced liver necrosis in mice by naturally occurring methylenedioxybenzenes. (Toxicol Appl Pharmacol, 1996 Oct)

Malaria

Rücker G, et al; Antimalarial activity of 1,4-epidioxy-bisabola-2,12-diene derivatives. (ArchPharm (Weinheim), 1997 Jan-Feb)

Respiratory System

Menon LG, et al; Inhibition of lung metastasis in mice induced by B16F10 melanoma cells by polyphenolic compounds. (Cancer Lett, 1995 Aug 16)

Polasa K, et al; Effect of turmeric on urinary mutagens in smokers. (Mutagenesis, 1992Mar)

Polasa K, et al; Turmeric (Curcuma longa)-induced reduction in urinary mutagens. (FoodChem Toxicol, 1991 Oct)

Srinivas L, et al; DNA damage by smoke: protection by turmeric and other inhibitors of ROS.(Free Radic Biol Med, 1991)

Venkatesan N, et al; Modulation of cyclophosphamide-induced early lung injury by curcumin, an anti-inflammatory antioxidant. (Mol Cell Biochem, 1995 Jan 12,)

Skin

Charles V, et al; The use and efficacy of Azadirachta indica ADR ('Neem') and Cur-

. t h e   s p i c e   o f   l i f e .

cumalonga ('Turmeric') in scabies. A pilot study. (Trop Geogr Med, 1992 Jan,)
Goh CL, et al; Allergic contact dermatitis to Curcuma longa (turmeric). (Contact Dermatitis,1987 Sep)
Hata M, et al; Allergic contact dermatitis from curcumin (turmeric). (Contact Dermatitis,1997 Feb)
Huang MT, et al; Inhibitory effects of topical application of low doses of curcumin on12-O-tetradecanoylphorbol-13-acetate-induced tumor promotion and oxidized DNA basesin mouse epidermis. (Carcinogenesis, 1997 Jan)
Iersel ML, et al; Inhibition of glutathione S-transferase activity in human melanoma cells byalpha,beta-unsaturated carbonyl derivatives. Effects of acrolein, cinnamalde-hyde, citral,crotonaldehyde, curcumin, ethacrynic acid, and trans-2-hexenal. (Chem Biol Interact, 1996Oct 21)
Ishizaki C, et al; Enhancing effect of ultraviolet A on ornithine decarboxylase induction anddermatitis evoked by 12-o-tetradecanoylphorbo l-13-acetate and its inhibition by curcuminin mouse skin. (Dermatology, 1996)
Kakar SS, et al; Curcumin inhibits TPA induced expression of c-fos, c-jun and c-mycproto-oncogenes messenger RNAs in mouse skin. (Cancer Lett, 1994 Nov 25, Abstractavailable)
Korutla L, et al; Inhibition of ligand-induced activation of epidermal growth factor receptortyrosine phosphorylation by curcumin. (Carcinogenesis, 1995 Aug)
Korutla L, et al; Inhibitory effect of curcumin on epidermal growth factor receptor kinaseactivity in A431 cells. (Biochim Biophys Acta, 1994 Dec 30)
Limtrakul P, et al; Inhibitory effect of dietary curcumin on skin carcinogenesis in mice.(Cancer Lett, 1997 Jun 24)
Lu YP, et al; Effect of curcumin on 12-O-tetradecanoylphorbol-13-acetate- and ultraviolet B light-induced expression of c-Jun and c-Fos in JB6 cells and in mouse epidermis.(Carcinogenesis, 1994 Oct)
Lu YP, et al; Inhibitory effect of curcumin on12-O-tetradecanoylphorbol-13-acetate-induced increase in ornithine decarboxylase mRNAin mouse epidermis. (Carcinogenesis, 1993 Feb)
Oda Y; Inhibitory effect of curcumin on SOS functions induced by UV irradiation. (MutatRes, 1995 Oct)
Suhaimi H, et al; Curcumin in a model skin lotion formulation. (J Pharm Sci, 1995 Mar)

Toxicity (lack of)

Abraham SK, et al; Genotoxicity of garlic, turmeric and asafoetida in mice. (Mutat Res, 1984Apr)
Abraham SK; Anti-genotoxic effects in mice after the interaction between coffee and dietaryconstituents. (Food Chem Toxicol, 1996 Jan)
Bille N, et al; Subchronic oral toxicity of turmeric oleoresin in pigs. (Food Chem Toxicol,1985 Nov)
Dahl TA, et al; Photocytotoxicity of curcumin. (Photochem Photobiol, 1994 Mar, Abstract available)

Jensen NJ; Lack of mutagenic effect of turmeric oleoresin and curcumin in theSal-monella/mammalian microsome test. (Mutat Res, 1982 Dec)

Kaphalia BS, et al; Organochlorine pesticide residues in different Indian cereals, pulses,spices, vegetables, fruits, milk, butter, Deshi ghee, and edible oils. (J Assoc Off Anal Chem,1990 Jul-Aug)

Shankar TN, et al; Toxicity studies on turmeric (Curcuma longa): acute toxicity studies inrats, guinea pigs & monkeys. (Indian J Exp Biol, 1980 Jan)

Worms

Jurgens TM, et al; Novel nematocidal agents from Curcuma comosa. (J Nat Prod, 1994Feb)

Kiuchi F, et al; Nematocidal activity of turmeric: synergistic action of curcuminoids. (ChemPharm Bull (Tokyo), 1993 Sep)

Womens' Reproductive System

Mehta RG, et al; Characterization of effective chemopreventive agents in mammary gland invitro using an initiation-promotion protocol. (Anticancer Res, 1991 Mar-Apr,)

Singh A, et al; Postnatal modulation of hepatic bio transformation system enzymes via translactational exposure of F1 mouse pups to turmeric and curcumin. (Cancer Lett, 1995Sep 4)

Singh AK, et al; Curcumin inhibits the proliferation and cell cycle progression of human umbilical vein endothelial cell. (Cancer Lett, 1996 Oct 1)

Singletary K, et al; Inhibition of 7,12-dimethylbenz[a]anthracene (DMBA)-induced mammary tumorigenesis and DMBA-DNA adduct formation by curcumin. (Cancer Lett, 1996 Jun 5)

Verma SP, et al; Curcumin and genistein, plant natural products, show synergistic inhibitory effects on the growth of human breast cancer MCF-7 cells induced by estrogenic pesticides.(Biochem Biophys Res Commun, 1997 Apr 28)